HIIT It!

HIIT It!

The Fitnessista's Get More from Less Workout and Diet Plan to Lose Weight and Feel Great Fast

Gina Harney

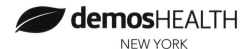

demosHEALTH

NEW YORK

Visit our website at www.demoshealth.com

ISBN: 978-1-936303-67-0
e-book ISBN: 978-1-617052-21-7

Acquisitions Editor: Julia Pastore
Compositor: diacriTech

Medical information provided by Demos Health, in the absence of a visit with a health care professional, must be considered as an educational service only. This book is not designed to replace a physician's independent judgment about the appropriateness or risks of a procedure or therapy for a given patient. Our purpose is to provide you with information that will help you make your own health care decisions.

The information and opinions provided here are believed to be accurate and sound, based on the best judgment available to the authors, editors, and publisher, but readers who fail to consult appropriate health authorities assume the risk of injuries. The publisher is not responsible for errors or omissions. The editors and publisher welcome any reader to report to the publisher any discrepancies or inaccuracies noticed.

Library of Congress Cataloging-in-Publication Data
   Harney, Gina.
   HIIT it! : the fitnessista's get more from less workout and diet plan to lose weight and feel great fast / Gina Harney.
      pages cm
   Includes bibliographical references and index.
   ISBN 978-1-936303-67-0
   1. Reducing exercises. 2. Reducing diets. 3. Physical fitness. 4. Weight training. 5. Weight loss.
6. Nutrition. I. Title.
   RA781.6.H355 2014
   613.7—dc23
                                2014027380

Special discounts on bulk quantities of Demos Health books are available to corporations, professional associations, pharmaceutical companies, health care organizations, and other qualifying groups. For details, please contact:

Special Sales Department
Demos Medical Publishing, LLC
11 West 42nd Street, 15th Floor
New York, NY 10036
Phone: 800-532-8663 or 212-683-0072
Fax: 212-941-7842
E-mail: specialsales@demosmedical.com

Printed in the United States of America by McNaughton & Gunn.
14 15 16 17 18 / 5 4 3 2 1

To Tom, Olivia, and my family for their love, support, and encouragement. I'm a lucky girl to have you in my life.

Contents

Being busy does not always mean real work. The object of all work is production or accomplishment and to either of these ends there must be forethought, system, planning, intelligence, and honest purpose, as well as perspiration.

—Thomas Edison

Preface

To all of my friends just getting started in fitness: Welcome to the start of a new and healthy lifestyle. I'm cheering for you every step of the way! Because you made the choice to be here, *you will succeed*. You have to want it for yourself to go after your goals, and by picking up this book, I hope you can find some useful tools to help you along your journey.

Although I am a certified group fitness instructor, personal trainer, and weight loss specialist, I'm not a medical doctor. It's within the scope of my knowledge and experience to make suggestions regarding healthy choices, portion control, and recipes; however, I am unable to make recommendations for special populations and unique needs. I enlisted the help of Anne Mauney to ensure that the meal and nutrition guidelines in this book are effective, safe, and align with general recommendations.

Anne Mauney, MPH, RD, is a Washington, DC, area registered dietitian with a Master's of Public Health in Nutrition from the University of North Carolina at Chapel Hill. Anne owns her own nutrition counseling private practice, through which she works with both virtual and in-person clients to help them to lose or maintain weight, feel healthier, and improve their relationships with food. She teaches clients how to eat intuitively, encouraging them to ditch the calorie counting diet mentality and enjoy whole, real foods (which includes dessert!). In addition to her client work, Anne is also the author of the healthy living and fitness blog fANNEtastic food (www.fannetasticfood.com), which she uses as a way to inspire readers to live happier, healthier lives through nutrition and exercise. On her blog, you'll find quick and easy meal ideas, simple healthy recipes, running training plans and adventures, and more.

To create the workout plans in this book, I thoroughly researched the most effective methods for combining strength and cardio into a solid routine to maximize your workout time. I send endless gratitude to Dr. Len Kravitz and Michael Zulh, MS, for their extensive research and studies regarding high-intensity interval training (HIIT). Their work encouraged me to expand my knowledge and understanding of HIIT, and I became a HIIT sponge, learning and experimenting as much as possible to share it with you. I hope this book can serve as your everything-HIIT resource and assist you in creating and changing the journey that starts right now.

Let's HIIT it, shall we?

As always, check with a doctor before making any fitness or nutrition changes. Honor your body and modify as needed.

Acknowledgments

Thank you so much to everyone who helped to make this book, and lifelong dream, a reality.

Special thanks to my agent, Chris Park, for your support, guidance, and tenacity over the past few years. You stuck with me through multiple proposals, concepts, and life changes along the way, and I couldn't be more appreciative.

To Julia Pastore, thank you for not only your editing prowess, but for being the one to initiate this incredible opportunity. It has been a pleasure to work with you on this book, and I'm filled with gratitude for your guidance and assistance along this journey.

Thanks to Lee Oglesby, Lucy Frisch, and the entire Demos Health team for bringing these pages to life.

Thanks to James Patrick for the beautiful photos. It's always an honor to work with you and I am so grateful for your expertise.

To Anne Mauney, thank you for your nutritional expertise and friendship "allthedays."

To my family, I am thankful for all of your love and support in my many endeavors. My nana and mom were always in the front row of my dance practices and recitals, and their cheers will remain in my heart while I tackle the many things I love and that I'm so grateful to do each day.

To Tom, my most valuable taste tester, behind-the-scenes blog editor, and love of my life; this book wouldn't have happened without you and your encouragement to stick with my goals.

Thanks to my military wife friends, especially Jeni, Ashley, Kelly, Jayme, Meara, Celia, Michelle, and Liz. You've been like sisters to me in this wild and crazy adventure, and I'm so thankful that the military world introduced me to all of you.

Thank you to Whitney "Whitters" who helped make San Diego instantly feel like home.

A special mention to my author friends who have inspired and supported me from afar: Matthew Kenney, who taught me the beauty and versatility of whole foods; Sarah Jio for your guidance and kindness; and Dreena Burton for inspiring me to creative, healthy, family-friendly recipes.

I'm always gracious to all of my blog friends, including but certainly not limited to: Meghann Anderson, Kasey Arena, Jenna Beaugh, Gabriela Benner, Carla Binberg, Theodora Blanchfield, Rebekah Borucki, Caitlin Boyle, Roo Ciambriello, Michelle Corso, Emma Cyders, Kelli Davis, Heather Demetra, Ashley Diamond, Sarah Dussault, Julie Fagan, Katie Gagliano, Sabrina Garibian, Danielle Hampton, Gena Hamshaw, Tina Haupert, Heather Hesington, Katie Higgins, Cassey Ho, Emily Holcombe Malone, Courtney Horan, Kacia Hosmer, TeriLyn Hutcheon, Janae Jacobs, Robyn Law, Angela Liddon, Sarah Matheny, Jessica Merchant, Bobbi McCormick, Ashley McLaughlin, Lori Morris, Erin Motzenbecker, Brittany Mullins, Katie O'Leary, Monica Olivas, Mara Rosenbloom, Liz Stark, Krisin Stehly, Averie Sunshine, Evan Thomas, Bethann Wagner, Sana Waheed, Maria Waldron, Katy Widrick and Kath Younger. I'm so blessed that the blog world introduced me to all of you, and honored to be part of an awesome group of virtual colleagues.

To all of my amazing blog readers. I am thankful for you each day. I created this book to share with all of you. Thank you for your support, for inviting my recipes to your kitchen table, taking my workouts to the gym with you, and for making the blog the inspiring community it has become. I hope you have as much fun reading this as I had creating it. Lots of love, healthy wishes, and boundless gratitude to you.

Introduction

At first glance, it can be easy to assume that someone has always had the same outward appearance and general disposition that he or she has now. There's no way to know someone's story without befriending them, and until then, it's easy to create visions in our mind of what that person's life may be like. Maybe it's just me, but I like to imagine the lives of perfect strangers (knowing that I'll be 100% inaccurate in my predictions). You never know the personal battles people may be experiencing, the steps they took to end up where they are right now, or the behind-the-scenes info on their lives: The mom I see at the bookstore, playing with her many kids who are all well-behaved, clean, and happy; she could have had a breakdown an hour before, and I'd have no idea. The man everyone knows at our gym, jovially walking around and killing it on the Smith machine; he's lost 100 pounds. And myself, a fitness instructor and blogger. Many years ago, I was a finance major at the University of Arizona. Fitness, a world I now know and love so dearly, was a foreign concept to me. I was overweight, uncomfortable in my own skin, and miserable.

My personal transformation story

During college, I taught dance classes to stay active, but I hadn't made the connection between food and body. Even though I had a lifestyle full of exercise (and walking all over campus to classes), I paired it with unhealthy eats. Over time, I could feel myself gaining weight, but wasn't sure what to do about it. In the sweltering Tucson summers, I wanted to wear cute tank tops, but when I looked in the mirror and saw my arms, I was self-conscious about showing them off. My weight eventually climbed to 40 pounds over a healthy range for my height. With lackluster skin and low energy, I knew something had to change, so I made the commitment to embark on a total lifestyle transformation.

The problem was that I knew I wanted to make some healthy changes, but I had no idea where to start. So I worked my way through the latest fad diets in succession. I'd start a new one when the current one would inevitably fail, thus beginning a long foray into yo-yo dieting. The first one was with the meal shakes. They were inexpensive (perfect for this then-college-girl's budget) and simple. I'd drink a shake instead of eating. I remember counting down the time until I could have my next shake, and I'd drink the powdery substance knowing that I didn't want to spend the rest of my life on a liquid (and HANGRY, which is hungry + angry) diet. Needless to say, it didn't last for very long.

Next, I was onto the low-carb (or no carb?!) thing. At first it worked fairly well, but since I'd lost mostly water weight, I gained some of it back when I tried to go back to eating normal foods. Just like the shakes, I knew it wouldn't be sustainable for the long term.

Eventually, I learned the beauty of Mediterranean eating, and for the first time I was making healthier choices, experimenting with new-to-me foods, and lost the extra weight while maintaining my energy. It was much easier for me to stick to, and through following this plan I learned how lean proteins, healthy fats, and smart carbs, could work together in harmony to aid my fat loss goals. It took about a year, and from that point, I've been able to maintain the 40 pounds I lost (except for that one time I gained it back to grow and birth a human).

At my new weight, I felt confident; clothes fit me the way nature intended instead of gathering, pinching, and sagging, and I had plenty of energy to make it through the day. My transformation changed me physically, but also mentally: my journey sparked a passion for health and fitness. I was determined to learn as much as possible about healthy living.

From then on, I was inspired to study fitness in conjunction with my undergraduate schoolwork. It became my hobby, and I was always interested to learn about new diet strategies or workout techniques. After I'd finish my homework for the evening, learning about fitness was my "dessert." During my last couple of years at college, I spent a lot of time at local coffee houses studying with friends. I guess fate was looking my way, because a certain coffee house was where I met my husband (whom I'll call the Pilot).

After that fateful night, I slowly watched my life entirely transform from what I'd been planning and imagined. Following graduation, and after making it through the Pilot's first deployment overseas, I packed up my belongings and moved with him to North Carolina. I quickly learned how difficult it is for a military spouse to become employed when you're moving so often. Since I had a finance degree, my first step was to try and use my degree in my profession. I applied to finance-related jobs, and I felt like the second a potential employer found out we were military, it was an invisible red "X" through my resume. Instead, I found a job in retail management, knowing it had nothing to do with my future goals.

I was unhappy with my job, living in a new place, away from family, and hadn't made friends yet. Fitness was the one thing I looked forward to each day. I woke up at 5:30 a.m. to get in a quick workout, and even though it was early (for me), I enjoyed getting in a sweat session before heading off to work. When I realized it was time for me to change paths and find a flexible job I enjoyed, fitness was the first thing to come to mind.

This realization was like a squat-jumping light bulb in my brain. Thinking about teaching fitness invigorated me, and when I drove down to Jacksonville to take my first certification exam, I knew I'd made the right choice. Becoming a fitness instructor would allow me to create an enjoyable path with my knowledge, and it was something I could continue to do with our constant moving and reassignments. Since then, the only use for my finance degree has been for our family budget and investments.

Too much, too far

Even though I was finally in maintenance mode as far as my personal weight goes, I had bigger goals on the fitness spectrum. I wanted to be LEAN, fitness modelesque, and eventually started to tack more and more onto my weight lifting and cardio routine. At one point, I was taking three fitness classes per day during the week (just typing that makes me shudder) and couldn't believe that I was so far away from where I wanted to be. Though I'd lost weight, I still had softness about my appearance. I failed to realize that I was eating away at the muscle

I'd created, which left me squishy … and I was spending too much time at the gym. When our calorie deficit is too high, this turns our muscles into hungry cannibals. They eat themselves, which is called muscular atrophy, and this contributes to the skinny–fat phenomenon I experienced.

Despite everything I'd learned over the past couple of years, I started to believe that "more was more" in terms of fitness. Instead of building precious lean muscle, I was earning it to burn it. This pattern continued on and off, bouts of insanely healthy eating paired with a quantity-over-quality mentality, until we moved back to Tucson and I began teaching at a world-renowned health resort.

More from less

One of my close fitness instructor friends had a mantra she would say throughout the day while we were teaching:

"Less is more. Less is more!"

We'd look at her side-eyed and laugh, because as fitness instructors, our bodies as our tools, we were jumping and burpeeing along with our classes. After the long day of teaching, we'd often find ourselves extremely run down from trying to keep up hour after hour. My wise instructor friend was the one leading by example, doing a few reps, and then walking around the class to coach. She was just as, if not more, motivational, and (bonus) she wasn't killing herself. I learned a lot from assisting her, and caught onto her strategy to get more effort from my classes without necessarily increasing active participation. "You do, you watch, you coach. Less is more. OK … unless it's Zumba. Then, MORE is MORE!!"

With fitness and healthy eating, I always thought more *was* more: more cardio was better; the more I could restrain myself from diving into a couple of brownies was better, right? So I did a ton of cardio, ate what I thought was as healthy as possible, and was disappointed to find my body light-years away from where I thought it should be with how hard I worked. I would spend an hour on the elliptical reading a magazine, and spent a lot of my time lifting weights. I stuck to virtually the same routine, and went through the motions I thought I needed to achieve the desired results I had set in my brain.

As time went on, I continued this failing fitness strategy. I would hear myself telling clients that nutrition is more important than workouts for fitness gains (this is TRUE!) and there I was, still logging significant cardio mileage and strength training in addition to the classes I taught. I was on an elliptical hamster ball to Nowheresville as far as dramatic change goes. Unknowingly, I was hindering any potential results through an extreme lifestyle I had mistaken for hard work. While I knew so much about fitness and how to incorporate strength and cardio, my Type A and slightly obsessive personality had me working too hard and taxing my body past its limit.

A few years later, my husband and I were blessed with our baby daughter. She's the best thing that's ever happened to our family, and has changed me in so many ways. With working on the blog, teaching classes, and my new job as a full-time mama, I didn't have time for the "more is more" mentality when it came to fitness and healthy eating. For the first year, I was exhausted and utilized a large portion of gym time for sleep, so I was lucky to get in a couple of sessions each week. Healthy eating also changed for me. Over my long stints with dieting and trying different things, I had also gotten into gluten-free, lower-carb, and packaged "health" foods. These weren't things I wanted my daughter to grow up eating, and I wanted her to know that no food is off limits. My stringent ways bit the dust. I started eating to fuel my body, aiming for quick and convenient meals so we could spend more time playing. It helped me to become more intuitive about eating—no more random snacking, and I made a point to eat when I was hungry—and I started to enjoy foods that I had dubbed "unhealthy" in years past and had nixed from my diet.

I wanted to teach my daughter the beauty of whole fresh foods, while enjoying treats and the "fun stuff" every now and again, too. We love homemade green juices, grilled fish, lovely smoothies, and sandwiches together, but we also have pizza nights, cookies, and have been known to hit up the bakery for some beautiful macaroons on a fairly regular basis. By endeavoring to teach my daughter to enjoy ALL foods, instead of labeling them as "good" or "bad," I myself found the balance I'd yearned so long to achieve. A *lifestyle*. I started to truly enjoy everything, and it was a giant sigh of relief that I could comfortably and easily maintain my fitness results. In the end, I weighed less and was a thousand times happier than I was on my hamster wheel: spending less time working out and no longer stressing about eating "perfectly" all the time. I've found that by being easier on myself, I didn't feel deprived and could more easily keep a healthy grand scheme of things. It doesn't have to be all or nothing; it truly is about finding that glorious balancing point with health, fitness, treats, and rest.

By making my workouts shorter yet more effective and relaxing my eating habits, I found my abs. This was by no means accidental—if it was, you would reach through this book and punch me ... I'd punch myself—but instead, I'd finally discovered how to get MORE with LESS. I figured out how to get the most from my lifestyle, more bang from my proverbial gym-time buck, and get the body I'd been working so hard to achieve. Along with the physical results, the most noticeable benefits occurred mentally: I felt more energized to keep up with the tasks at hand, and I had a higher sense of clarity and presence.

I'm sure many of you have found yourselves in a similar situation, daunted and afraid to make changes, or maybe on the other end of the spectrum, by doing way too much in hopes of quicker results. An event or realization can shift the priority totem pole, and you eventually reach a breaking point. You don't want to be unhealthy any longer. You determine you need to change up your routine. Or you find you're doing way too much in a manner that isn't sustainable for the long-term.

With my newfound duties as a mama, I had to dramatically shift my fitness schedule, and in doing so, I learned how to make my workouts and healthy eating truly work for me. Now, I focus on my family, my friends, my work, and see healthy cuisine and fitness as fun hobbies. They no longer take over my life, they now complement and facilitate all of the things I love to do. This was the beginning of the HIIT lifestyle: High Intensity Interval Training paired with Healthy, Intuitive, Intermittent meals, and Tracked eats. After simplifying my routine and making my strategies the most effective they've ever been, I'm never going back to the drudgery of the past. By doing more (and more, and more ...), the fun was sucked out of things I originally enjoyed so much. By reducing my gym time while increasing creativity in my workouts and the kitchen, it revitalized my love for healthy living.

Utilizing strategies from the extremely popular HIIT, I translated the methodology to my diet. With HIIT, you're working as hard as possible for a short amount of time, and then reaping the rewards throughout the day. That's the same thing I'm doing with my eating: maximum effort for a short period of time (by planning and prepping lots of clean eats for the week ahead), and enjoying the results with a constant stream of fresh, whole choices on hand throughout the week. Just like cardio and training, we need to alternate our eating intensities and intake. Our body is an intelligent machine that will kick into cruise control when imposed with the same demands, so by constantly changing things up, we force it to change along with us. For this reason, I'm constantly changing my nutrient intake to keep my body guessing, all while enjoying foods I truly love.

In my fitness routine, I'm no longer spending more than 40 minutes working out, unless I'm teaching/taking a class. If I teach a class that day, it's counted as my workout—no more extra gym time for this girl. The same goes for many of you. If you spend the day doing something extremely active (gardening, dance party with the kiddos, walking around while exploring a new city), you don't need to spend the extra time at the gym. Utilizing circuit training, high intensity intervals, steady state, balance, and flexibility, I've created short yet effective schedules, maximizing efficiency and streamlining my routine. They're all included in this book, along with ways to spice up your workout schedule, keep your body guessing, and avoid plateaus.

I'll also go over all of the details for effective eating strategies (pre- and postworkout, planning for the week, and the HIIT style of eating) and explain everything I had to learn the hard way. By splitting your food into general macronutrient categories (P = protein, F = fat, C = carb, N = neutral, T = treat), it's much easier to create fat-burning and satisfying combos, while enabling you to stick to a lifestyle you can enjoy and maintain. Quick fixes mean short-term results. I hope this book helps you create a personalized workout and healthy eating plan with satisfying results and long-term staying power. The key to success is consistency.

This isn't a "diet" book. This isn't a workout book. Though I hope you find new diet strategies and tons of new workouts, the goal is to help you create the best *lifestyle* for YOU. You'll be able to easily maintain, enjoy all of the glorious things in life, and reap the benefits of your work. That being said, there is no one-size-fits-all recommendation for a diet and fitness plan. In this book are strategies that have worked for past and currents clients and the most nagging, demanding client I have—myself. I hope you find these tips and strategies helpful, and learn how to get more from less. If there's one thing we all have in common, it's that we're busy. There's no need to overcomplicate things, reinvent the wheel, or pedal along in a hamster ball to Nowheresville.

HIIT to fit, baby.

Part One

HIIT It! Fitness

Chapter 1

HIIT Training 101

High intensity interval training (HIIT) is one of the most popular current training techniques. This strategy, alternating bouts of extreme effort and recovery periods, is one of the fastest and most effective cardiovascular training methods. The health and fitness world has caught on to its effectiveness and overwhelmingly positive results, thus becoming a huge trend in the fitness industry. Unlike many "Hollywood" workout fads that lack scientific backing or long-term sustainability, HIIT is here to stay. Its short duration coupled with high effectiveness makes it an ideal workout for busy people. Even though HIIT is currently the hottest of the hot, it has been around much longer than many of us may realize. Can you believe successful athletes have used this training technique for over a century? The first recorded usage of HIIT was in 1912, but let's be real: you know cavemen unintentionally did HIIT intervals while sprinting from predators.

The first recorded HIIT athletes (distance runners and endurance athletes) utilized this training strategy to improve their performance, and almost all of the Olympic medalists of the early 1900s attributed their success to some type of interval training. So, while HIIT has a proven track record (pun?) as a quick and effective way to achieve fitness results and fat loss, it can be slightly intimidating to implement without a little guidance. Here's a little HIIT 101 for those of you who are just learning, as well as for seasoned vets that could benefit from a review of the basics.

The "skinny" on HIIT

HIIT is a cardiovascular technique of short bouts of extreme effort followed by rest. HIIT workouts are quick and dirty, never lasting more than 30 minutes (including warm-up and short cool-down). You can perform these intervals with any mode of cardio such as biking, jumping rope, running, rowing, stair-climbing, or by doing plyometrics (power movements requiring muscles to exert maximum force in minimal time), or calisthenics (using your own bodyweight as resistance). The length of time spent exercising can be adjusted according to your personal fitness level. An advanced exerciser is capable of shorter periods of rest with higher effort and longer intervals of exercising, while a beginner would exercise with lower intensity and longer bouts of rest between interval sets.

Examples:

Beginner: 1:2 ratio of work and rest, that is, 30 seconds hard, 1 to 2 minute rest; repeat as many times as possible within a 10 to 15 minute set.

Intermediate: 1:2 ratio of work and rest, or equal work-to-rest ratios, that is, 30 seconds hard, 30 second to 1 minute rest; repeat as many times as possible within a 15 to 20 minute set.

Advanced: Equal work-to-rest ratio or double work-to-rest ratio, that is, 30 seconds hard, 15 to 30 second rest; repeat as many times as possible within a 20 to 25 minute set.

From here, you can play with the interval sets and increase the amount of rest time or work once you get comfortable within a certain set. In other words, if 30 seconds starts to feel too easy, you can increase the duration (no longer than two minutes) or increase your work capacity. The goal is to push yourself during your working zones, so whether you need to do that by speed, increasing range of motion (changing the height dynamic or adding a jump is an easy way to do this), or adding some resistance through a higher incline or using light weights, it's up to you. Challenge yourself safely and according to your personal fitness level.

Between intervals, you should feel your heart rate come back down to a recovery zone. If you're going by perceived exertion, during the hard bouts of effort you should not be able to speak more than two words in a sentence ("THIS! SUCKS!"). During recovery you should be able to spit out a three to four word sentence ("OK. It's. Over. That. Rocked!"). *Your work should feel like work; your rest should feel like an easy recovery*. Remember that by pushing yourself you don't need to work as *long*, if you focus. Just remember, you're already making the effort; now make it count!

If you're using a heart rate monitor, use the formulas below to calculate your interval heart rates:

Your Maximum Heart Rate	
220 − [Your Age]	Example: 30-year-old woman 220 − 30 = 190 Maximum Heart Rate is 190
Your Recovery Zone	
60%–70% of your Maximum Heart Rate	Example: 190 × .60 = 114 190 × .70 = 133 Recovery Zone is 114–133
Your Work Zone	
80%–95% of your Maximum Heart Rate	Example: 190 × .80 = 152 190 × .95 = 181 Work Zone is 152–181

Both the speed of your heart rate drop and the amount of that decrease during your recovery indicate that your heart is beginning to work more effectively. If you notice that you're in a recovery zone and start to feel like you're ready to HIIT it again before the official interval begins, you can play with decreasing the recovery time and/or increasing the work intervals.

A word about diminishing returns: Don't automatically assume that higher is better as far as your heart rate goes. Once you're in the working anaerobic zone, you are seeing fairly equal benefits to those you would if maxing out your heart rate entirely. Just focus on making it to the point where you feel as if you're working hard, but not that you wouldn't be able to do more than one interval at that speed and capacity. After a certain point you may start to see diminishing returns, especially if you work out too hard, too quickly. It's not worth injuring yourself, right? PS: Even though people are usually too wrapped up in their own workout to notice what other people are doing, interval training is hard to miss. To everyone passing by as you train, you look hardcore no matter how fast you're going; they just see you interval training and working hard. Who knows? They may be inspired to add some energy bursts and challenge themselves during their own future workout sessions.

Also, don't equate modifications or rest with weakness. You need a solid rest interval in order to classify the routine as true interval training. By failing to include proper rest, not only are you robbing yourself of excess benefits (with a solid rest interval, you're able to push it even harder and get more out of your work intervals), but you will set your-self up for increased risk of adaptation, injury, and burnout. HIIT is a valuable fitness tool, but it should be used responsibly and correctly in order to maximize the rewards.

A few benefits of HIIT training

HIIT training makes maintaining a steady state easier, and can boost power in your normal workout routines. When you're used to maintaining the same effort for the duration of your workout, the bursts of energy and effort required for HIIT will make your steady state feel like a breeze. According to a 2013 study in the *European Journal of Sport Science*, two groups of cyclists were assigned to either long bouts of high-intensity intervals or shorter-duration intervals. Both groups had similar biophysical results (an increase of 7% in peak oxygen, which indicates improved fitness), but the long-interval group was able to significantly decrease their 5K run time. This is a good indication that it's beneficial to alternate the types and durations of intervals you perform. The benefits of interval training translate across a variety of fitness modalities and are similar to those of longer endurance training in just a fraction of the time.

HIIT can help fight the urge to snack. High-intensity training can affect our appetites following a session. According to a recent study by the *Journal of Obesity*, subjects demonstrated reduced appetite following HIIT training. I've noticed in my own experience that *any* type of fitness training will also affect the quality of foods I choose for my body. I feel more inspired to eat whole, healthy foods when I've had a great exercise session. My body also requires more hydration following a workout, so I'm naturally inclined to reach for foods with a high water content, such as fresh fruits and veggies. Dense and low-nutrient foods such as sugary snacks and greasy starches sound dramatically less appealing when I'm sweaty and my body seeks hydration, protein (for muscle recovery), and smart carbohydrate to replenish my energy stores.

If you work to make it count, you'll get the same results as if you'd worked out longer with less intensity. In 2007 research by the *American Journal of Human Biology*, exercise participants were divided into two groups: one for HIIT and the other for moderate intensity. The results of the study were similar for both groups, but the moderate-intensity group exercised for 420 minutes during the seven-week study, while the HIIT group only trained for 63 minutes (about 15%!). When you're performing HIIT, you're working out SMARTER, not longer.

HIIT utilizes different aerobic pathways, muscular functions, and internal motivation techniques. The sprinting and jumping movements often used in HIIT training will also help to improve leg strength, coordination, agility, and balance, which is especially important as we age. HIIT training, especially in addition to a solid strength routine, will also help to foster healthy bone density, create lean muscle, and protect our joints over time. When you complete a tough interval workout, it requires intense internal motivation to convince yourself to work as hard as possible. Your body becomes fatigued, but it seems as if the mind is always the first to quit. By motivating yourself to keep going, especially during something so challenging, you are creating internal motivation and drive that will help in all of your day-to-day tasks and activities.

By spiking your heart rate up and then allowing it to come back down to a resting or recovery state before elevating it again, *you are training your heart to work more efficiently.* In doing so, you're able to burn a high amount of calories fairly quickly. HIIT sessions of just 13 minutes can burn as many calories as a 40-minute low-intensity session, according to a January 2014 study by *Medicine & Science in Sports & Exercise.* A major contributor to this phenomenon is called excess postexercise oxygen consumption (EPOC). When you perform endurance cardio at a low to moderate intensity—let's say a longer run—the calories expended during the workout are basically the total amount you can expect to burn from your efforts. After a HIIT workout, you continue to burn more calories throughout the day as your body works to restore your preworkout oxygen levels.

EPOC is affected by the duration and intensity of the training load. After exercise, the body must use increased oxygen to restore the body to a resting state by replenishing energy supplies and lowering tissue temperature. This means that in doing so, it's burning more calories than it was before the exercise was initiated. A pleasant surprise: you're efficiently burning fat throughout the day, even while you're working at your desk or lounging with your favorite TV show. *The higher the intensity of the workout, the greater the magnitude of EPOC.* Splitting training sessions throughout the day increases EPOC even more, because instead of one, you'll have multiple EPOC sessions. This is a huge advantage for those who aren't able to complete a longer workout in a single bout; split it up and reap the EPOC rewards. Another bonus: if you split up your workout, you may have more energy to work harder each time, so don't fret if you don't have a large time block during the day to devote to exercise.

HIIT is a fat-burning machine. HIIT training also increases the size and amount of mitochondria in our cells, which are the fat-burning fires of our metabolism. In a 2007 study, seven sessions of HIIT over a 2-week period induced marked increases in whole body and skeletal muscle capacity for fatty acid oxidation during exercise in moderately active women. Each session consisted of 10 four-minute bouts at 90% of their VO2 max (maximal oxygen consumption), with two minutes of rest between intervals. These women were able to increase their body fat oxidation by 36% following their HIIT workouts.

This is something that I've also witnessed in my own fitness routine and while training clients. Women have come in to see me after following a solid steady-state cardio routine, basic strength training, and relatively clean eats. They still have fitness and fat loss goals they'd like to accomplish. We add in strategic HIIT training, and *BAM*! It pushes them out of stagnation to where they want to be. Interval training is also what helped me lean out after having my baby. I didn't have a lot of time to dedicate to my workouts, so when I did cardio, it was usually intervals.

In the process, HIIT also decreases abdominal fat. Can I get an "ohhh yeah!" from everyone out there? HIIT training has been demonstrated to reduce subcutaneous (aka stubborn and deep) abdominal fat, as well as reducing insulin resistance. Many HIIT training techniques also encourage core strength, which is beneficial for posture, balance, and preventing back ailments.

Some differences between HIIT and steady state

Obviously, *HIIT workouts are shorter.* After a warm-up at moderate pace, the body of the workout should range from 15 to 30 minutes max. After 30 minutes, you shouldn't be able to continue to do intervals if you're working at max capacity. Work out harder and smarter, not longer. There are always ways to increase the difficulty of your HIIT workouts without increasing the duration.

HIIT workouts are fun and exciting. OK, so "fun" can be a bit of a reach, but you won't feel bored while you're doing a HIIT workout. Often, you'll notice that the session goes by extremely fast! It can be so invigorating that you'll actually be sad that it's over. Steady-state workouts, however, last significantly longer and can feel monotonous over time. This is another reason why it's important to include a solid mix in your training routine, which is exactly what's offered in the workouts in the following chapters. Variety is the spice of life (and the secret to avoiding plateaus).

Steady state is an entirely different beast. Think of a steady-state workout as a long run, spin class (which may incorporate intervals), dance class, or a fast-paced walk. Steady state helps to increase aerobic endurance, which is beneficial for our cardiovascular and muscular systems. In a steady-state workout, you'll burn a significant amount of calories, and this cardio option is something that can be done every day. Steady-state training is also a more appropriate option for beginners. If you're just getting started with a fitness routine or bouncing back from an injury (with a doctor's "OK" to begin or resume exercise), endeavor to build up your cardio base before experimenting with intervals. You should be able to easily complete 30 minutes of steady-state cardio most days of the week (at a moderate intensity) before attempting any type of interval work.

A solid fitness routine includes HIIT and steady-state components

HIIT training challenges both your aerobic and anaerobic systems (that is, using oxygen and without using oxygen as fuel). While HIIT is beneficial for building speed and power, steady state can help to increase endurance. If you look at these types of training from a functional perspective, you need a balance of power (to lift, sprint, jump, etc.) and endurance (to hike, walk, perform activities on your feet all day) to make it through daily motions without an increased chance of injury.

Benefits that both techniques share

According to studies by Len Kravitz and Michael Zuhl, here are some benefits that HIIT and continuous endurance training have in common:

- *Improved cardiac output through increased stroke volume (which improves oxygen transport to the working muscles), increased cardiac muscle mass, and function of the left ventricle.* By increasing proper function of our cardiac system, we lower the risk of heart-related health complications.

- *Increased metabolism,* through an increase in oxidative enzymes and mitochondria. Our metabolism is able to work more efficiently to burn fat.

- *Higher fat oxidation.* Any type of cardiovascular exercise will promote fat oxidation.

- *Faster diffusion of oxygen and fuel into muscle.* This is an indication of improved fitness and efficiency!

- *Higher expression of slow-twitch muscle fibers.* Our slow twitch (Type I) muscles are more efficient at using oxygen to generate fuel for muscle contractions lasting a long time, as in a long run or bike ride. They fire more slowly than Type II (fast twitch) muscle fibers and are slower to fatigue. By higher expression of these muscle groups, we're encouraging faster endurance fitness gains.

- *Increased disposal of metabolic waste.* If our body is able to take out the proverbial trash more effectively, that means it's then able to perform other critical tasks without being bogged down by digestive and detoxification processes.

Steady-state and HIIT cardio are both extremely beneficial for fat loss and fitness gains in their own way. By changing it up, not only are you reducing your chance of overuse injuries and burnout, but you'll also feel more balanced, invigorated, and physically powerful with a routine incorporating both cardio methods. If you'd like to incorporate HIIT in your routine, here are some tips and guidelines to follow.

Before you HIIT it

- Talk with a doctor before making any fitness or nutrition changes.

- HIIT workouts should be challenging, but they should never be painful. If you start to feel pain (especially in your legs or chest), STOP. Never push it to the point of pain. Remember that you can always progress your workout to make things more challenging, or modify to accommodate for specific considerations.

- Always warm up at a moderate pace and intensity for 5 to 10 minutes before completing a HIIT workout.

- Never perform HIIT training on consecutive days. High-intensity intervals utilize our heart to its maximum capacity. Our heart is a muscle—I'd say the most important one!—and needs time to rest and recover, just like any other muscles (biceps, triceps, leg, etc.).

- Remember that results occur during *rest*, so this is why it's crucial to alternate cardio intensities and facilitate recovery.

- Before completing a HIIT workout, you should be able to easily complete 30 minutes of moderate-intensity steady-state cardio (70%–85% of your maximum heart rate, which is 220 minus your age. For example, if you're 30 years old, this would be $220 - 30 = 190 \times .70 = 133$ for the heart rate floor and $190 \times .85 = 161.5$ for the ceiling; for this example, you'd want your heart rate to be in the range of 133 to 165 beats per minute).

(continued)

■ If you have any health considerations or doubts concerning your perceived ability to complete a HIIT workout, consult with a medical professional. When beginning a new fitness plan of any type, talk with your doctor to get his or her approval and/or advice regarding modifications

Word to the wise: start easy and work up from there. It's safer for your body to do something that's too easy and move up, than to overtax and over exhaust your system, which is a quick ticket to injury city. You know your body and its limits; it's up to you to pay attention and listen to what your body is telling you. You can always modify according to your unique needs. Remember, if you change *anything*, your body will respond. There's no need to go all crazypants from the get-go. Build up.

Some advice for beginners

HIIT is not recommended for fitness beginners or those with heart concerns or hip, knee, and/or joint considerations. Check with your doctor before beginning any type of fitness plan, and honor your body.

That being said, there are some ways to utilize HIIT strategies in your beginning fitness plan, as well as some low-impact HIIT options:

■ *You don't need to go balls to the wall.* If you're an advanced or intermediate exerciser with a strong fitness foundation, you will be able to push yourself during the interval sets. If you're just starting out, make sure you can comfortably complete 30 minutes of steady-state cardio, five days per week, before experimenting with speed surges. Beginners: If you go for a 30-minute walk or jog five days each week, you are still working your cardiovascular system, improving fitness, and burning calories! After you feel comfortable with that, you can talk to a doc about incorporating interval training.

■ *Aim for shorter work intervals with longer periods of rest.* A great starting point is 20 to 30 seconds of more challenging effort and two minutes of rest. Alternate for a shorter workout (10 to 15 total minutes to start; increase time or decrease intervals as this becomes easier). After you become more comfortable with the idea of adding intervals or speed surges, you can start to increase the work duration or decrease the rest duration.

- *For low-impact options, experiment with joint-friendly modes, including the spin bike, elliptical, and swimming.* The spin bike is an excellent starting point for interval training. Many classes incorporate speed drills and tempo work, which is fantastic for increasing your heart rate and bringing it back down to a recovery state.

It's funny because back in the day, I thought the spin bike looked "so easy." (Keep in mind that I do not know how to ride a real bike.) My first spin class made me eat my words ... my roommates almost had to carry me up the stairs to our apartment the next day! The beauty of spinning is that you can decrease or increase the work depending on your fitness level and experience, but keep in mind that you may be a liiiiitle sore and walking funny after the first time.

- Jogging in the pool is another wonderful low-impact cardio option, whether you run while pumping water weights or utilizing an underwater treadmill. Many gyms offer aqua fitness classes that are very easy on the joints, especially if you've recently recovered from an injury. When you're taking aqua classes, remember that you have the additional resistance of the water, so the bigger and faster the movements are, the more challenging it will be. Use your entire foot on the pool floor—it can be tempting to "tippy toe" the entire time—and enjoy the change of scenery! Just like spin classes, I had no idea how challenging water workouts could be when I first did them. I think it's just like anything: you get out of it what you put into it.

- *For bodyweight cardio options and plyometrics: beginners should keep one foot on the floor at all times.* Avoid jumping and experiment with range of motion instead. For example, during a squat jump, you would reach toward the floor (squat) and come up onto your tiptoes with arms extended overhead. This will increase your heart rate significantly without the necessity of joint impact.

■ *A simple way to make an exercise simultaneously easier and more challenging: slow down.* I think many of us have a perceived notion that faster is better, but maintaining proper form is far more important than speed. I'd rather see 10 beautiful squats than 100 cringeworthy attempts for the sake of obtaining a certain repetition amount. When you sacrifice form for speed, not only are you knocking at injury's door, but you could also be cheating yourself of a more effective workout. Concentrate on the muscles you're working as you move with intention through the exercise.

Incorporating HIIT intervals into your routine

To get the most out of your HIIT workouts, there are a few ways to include them in your routine. Here are a couple of options:

1) *Strength* and *HIIT (or the other way around).* There are mixed opinions about whether you should complete the cardio or strength portion of your workout first. My belief: assess your goals and go from there. You will likely have more energy for the first portion of your workout and be able to work harder. So if fat burning is your goal, I suggest performing the cardio or HIIT portion of your workout first. If strength gain and building lean muscle is your primary goal, do your strength set first and follow it with cardio. At the end of the day, personal preference is key. The combo doesn't make a huge difference; going to the gym and completing your workout is going to have the higher impact on success. The best workout is the one you'll *do.*

2) *HIIT blasts intertwined with your strength sets.* A successful HIIT method is to perform a short round of HIIT intervals between your strength training sets. This will blast your heart rate and enable you to burn more calories during your workout, as your

heart rate will be elevated during the strength portions. (Also, if you perform circuit training, moving quickly from one exercise to the next, this will help to maintain a higher heart rate during the workout.) For this method, perform a few sets of your strength exercises and add a cardio blast for 30 seconds to one minute before repeating the strength circuit or moving on to the next set of exercises. (For example, if you're doing a circuit of squats, pull-ups, and push-ups, go through one set of each exercise, add in one minute of squat jumps and then repeat the circuit of squats, pull-ups, and push-ups before squat jumping again.)

3) *HIIT and steady state.* This is one of my all-time favorite HIIT methods. You'll perform HIIT intervals at any ratio (all thoroughly explained in chapter 2), and combine this with easy steady-state cardio. This will teach your body to effectively burn fat, and also make your regular steady-state workouts feel much easier. It's also fun to add up to five minutes of HIIT intervals to the end of a long run, or as the grand finale after any long, steady-state cardio session.

Common HIIT mistakes

- *Making the rest intervals too short or the work intervals too long.* As I said before, start easy and work your way up from there.

- *Performing HIIT on consecutive days.* Give your body time to rest and repair; be sure to alternate cardio intensities. Don't work out at the same intensity as you did yesterday. For me, an ideal week of workouts includes three really challenging days, two moderate days, one easy day, and one off day.

- *Choosing exercises that will not get your heart rate up in a short amount of time.* I've seen some HIIT videos that have regular ol' biceps curls as the "work" ratios. Nope. Choose something that will challenge your cardiovascular system quickly, so you don't have to wait until rep 12 for it to kick in.

Here are some of my all-time favorite HIIT methods, research-backed for the best results.

Sample HIIT workouts

HIIT 1:1 ratios (distance or time)

1:1 ratios involve using either the same time set for rest and work, or the same distance. For example, you'll do one minute hard and one minute easy, or .25 miles hard, .25 miles easy. The work and rest ratios are equal, and sandwiched between a proper warm-up and cool-down.

Here are some examples, increasing in difficulty. Warm up and cool down adequately.

HIIT 1:1 Ratios
15–25 minutes max
2 minutes hard yet maintainable effort   2 minutes rest
1 minute hard   1 minute rest
30 seconds hard   30 seconds rest
1 mile challenging yet maintainable effort   1 mile easy
.50 mile hard   .50 mile easy
.25 mile hard   .25 mile easy

HIIT 2:1 ratios (distance or time)

Very similar to the 1:1 ratio method, but you'll double the work load and half the rest load. As you can probably guess, this is a more challenging method than the 1:1 ratio.

Here are some examples, increasing in difficulty. Warm up and cool down adequately.

HIIT 2:1 Ratios
15–25 minutes max
2 minutes hard yet maintainable effort 1 minute rest
1 minute hard 30 seconds rest
30 seconds hard 15 seconds rest
1 mile challenging yet maintainable effort .50 mile easy
.50 mile hard .25 mile easy

HIIT and Steady State

This is one of the *best* ways to lose fat. You'll complete your HIIT set using any of the methods above. For the same amount of time as your HIIT set, you'll complete easy steady state (50% of your max heart rate).

Here are some examples, increasing in difficulty. Warm up and cool down adequately:

HIIT and Steady State
10 minutes HIIT
10 minutes steady
15 minutes HIIT
15 minutes steady
20 minutes HIIT
20 minutes steady
25 minutes HIIT
25 minutes steady

Pyramid HIIT

For this method, you'll increase the time or distance of your work phase during the set. You can play with the recovery ratio, but I prefer to keep the recovery time the same for each round (it's less confusing this way). Go up to your highest time or distance amount, then come back down the pyramid following the same method.

Here are some time examples, increasing in difficulty. Warm up and cool down adequately:

Pyramid HIIT, time
15 seconds hard
30 seconds rest

30 seconds hard
30 seconds rest
1 minute hard
30 seconds rest
2 minutes hard
30 seconds rest
30 seconds hard
30 seconds rest
1 minute hard
30 seconds rest
1 minute 30 seconds hard
30 seconds rest
2 minutes hard
30 seconds rest
30 seconds hard
30 seconds rest
1 minute hard
1 minute rest
2 minutes hard
2 minutes rest

Here is a distance example. Warm up and cool down adequately:

Pyramid HIIT, distance
.10 mile hard
.25 mile rest
.5 mile hard
.25 mile rest
1 mile rest
.25 mile rest
.5 mile hard
.25 mile rest
.10 mile hard
.25 mile rest

Hill and Speed HIIT

This is one of my favorite methods of HIIT training ("favorite" is subjective). For this one, you'll be playing with resistance in addition to speed. You'll increase resistance, maintaining your speed, and then as the resistance is decreased, the speed goes up. It's a lot of fun, I promise.

Hill and Speed HIIT		
Time	Incline	Speed
0:00–5:00	2.0%	Fast walk or slow jog; you're warming up
5:00–10:00	Add 0.5%–1.0% every 30 seconds	Maintain your speed

10:00–12:00	Maintain your highest resistance	Maintain your speed
12:00–22:00	Decrease 1.0% every minute	Increase your speed by at least .2 mph
22:00–25:00	2.0%	Fast (run or power walk)
25:00–30:00	2.0%	Cool down. Slow and easy

Your budget-friendly HIIT home gym

One of the most appealing benefits about HIIT is the fact that you can do it anywhere with a limited amount of space and your own body weight. Check out the fitness photo sections of the book for heart-pounding cardio moves utilizing body weight alone.

If you have a small space you'd like to dedicate to your home gym, here are some tips for accomplishing this in a cost-friendly manner.

Building a home gym can be a daunting yet very fun adventure. With any big project, I tend to get in over my head, and thankfully the Pilot can rein me back in to reality. When the wheels in my brain started scheming our home gym, I imagined the super swanky "home gyms" from reality TV. As glorious as it would be, I knew a couple of things: there was no way we were making that kind of investment, and there was also no way I could convince the husband to fully convert his man cave to a fitness facility. Something that helped convince him: I built a fully functional home gym in our garage, complete with a spin bike and gym flooring, for less than $400.

Cardio

Pick a cardio option that you know you'll enjoy and do often. For this one, the investment can range from a free run around your neighborhood to a $3,000 treadmill. Evaluate your budget and determine how much you'd like to dedicate to your cardio investment. Some options: a fitness jump rope (fantastic for intervals), treadmill, indoor rower, spin bike, or plyometric blocks. I don't recommend ellipticals as they're not the most functional piece of fitness equipment. When in your life are you prancing around making oval-esque shapes with your feet? Ellipticals were originally intended for rehabilitation purposes before becoming popular fitness equipment. I only recommend frequent elliptical use if you're recovering from an injury. (A little note: from a training standpoint, I feel as if there are some more functional and effective options out there. If you love your elliptical and it is the only cardio you will consistently do, rock on with your bad self and enjoy!)

Freebie cardio

Bodyweight plyometrics. Burpees, butt kicks, high knees, jumping lunges, squat jumps, jogging in place, and basketball throws will get your heart rate up quickly while providing cardiovascular and fitness benefits. There are low-impact versions too, if you're trying to mini-mize joint pounding. The key is to create height and level dynamics without impact. Try reaching for the floor, bending your knees into a deep squat and standing up quickly, reaching your arms up toward the ceiling and coming onto your tip toes. Repeat quickly—you'll be surprised at how fast it can elevate your heart rate.

Jump rope. Your only expense is the cost of the jump rope (around $10) and you can get a killer *Rocky*-style cardio workout at home. (Bonus: you don't have to chase after any chickens.) My favorite method is to do intervals (of course) with 15 seconds on, 15 seconds rest, for 20 minutes. It looks easy on paper, but you will be drenched in sweat! The short intervals make the session fly by, and you can also get fancy with cross-country feet, double unders, or high knees as you jump rope.

Outdoor running. If you have a nearby track or safe spot in your neighborhood to run or walk briskly, this is one of the most effective types of freebie cardio. To add in strength blitzes, you can stop every couple of minutes to do some push-ups, tricep dips, walking lunges, burpees, or a plank. No one will think you're weird … just awesome. The three main tools for an effective strength and cardio workout are determination, a solid plan, and your own body weight.

Strength

Every home gym needs at least one solid form of strength equipment. Bodyweight strength exercises are fantastic for building lean muscle, but you can only challenge yourself to a certain point. You always want to impose additional challenges to your body during your fitness activities, and after the bodyweight movements become too easy, you have two options: increase the amount of repetitions, or increase the intensity through a more challenging option (example: push-ups on your toes instead of your knees) or additional resistance from an external source. Some ideas:

Tubing (aka resistance bands). These are a great low-cost option and are ideal for travel and smaller spaces, as they're light and don't take up much room. You can also purchase a door attachment to affix to a closed door for pushing and pulling movements, such as chest presses and rows.

Dumbbells. The classic never dies. While they're on the relatively expensive side, a dumbbell set can be a worthwhile investment. If you don't want to commit to an entire set, try picking up two pairs of dumbbells: a light set for smaller muscle groups (including triceps and shoulders) and a heavy set for the larger muscle groups (for example, bent-over rows and weighted squats). When these weights become too easy, many second-hand equipment stores will enable you to get a trade-in credit toward your next set(s).

Kettlebells. These are the most expensive option, but make a fantastic multipurpose strength component. Kettlebells have a unique center of gravity, which forces you to stabilize your core while you're working with them. Of course, invest in kettlebells once you have experience with a certified coach and you're looking to change things up from dumbbells.

> Don't skimp on strength training. I like to say that cardio will help to "shrink" your body, but weight training is going to have the most impact on shape and muscle density. Endeavor to create a balance of strength, cardio, core, flexibility, and balance training.

Flexibility and extras

Foam roller. I like to say "It Hurts So Good" (OK, and sing the song) while I foam roll, as it can get a little intense. I've seen grown men cry while foam rolling. See the appended section on foam rolling tips starting on page 305.

(continued)

A mat. This isn't necessary—a towel works just as well—but is nice for at-home yoga practices and stretching. There are options ranging from $10 to $100+, so find one that works for you and your lifestyle. If you practice yoga regularly (or would like to), a more expensive mat can be worth the investment, but if you're going to use it for stretching and at-home exercises, a less expensive option is a recommended starting point.

Chin-up bar. This is my secret weapon for chiseled arms, and let's be real, I can't even do a ton of chin-ups. When I was first learning how to do these, I'd place a sturdy chair underneath the chin-up bar. I'd stand on the chair, get into position, and lift one leg off the chair as I performed the movements. This way, it was more of an assisted pull-up and I didn't have to go from zero to straight pull-up power without working my way up. Pull-ups and chin-ups are a fantastic way to work your lat muscles and biceps, plus they can double as a core workout. I'll hang from the pull-up bar and do leg raises, bent knee tucks, and windshield wipers (bent knees, rotating my legs side to side). They're about $20 and easy to install in any doorway.

Stretching straps. These are wonderful for at-home yoga practice if you're just starting to work on your flexibility. A little tip: I recommend taking a couple of studio classes if you're just getting started with yoga. Just like strength training, it's helpful to get form cues and tips from a pro before venturing out on your own.

Chapter 2

HIIT to Fit

So now that we know what HIIT training is, here's how to incorporate this training technique into your own routine. While you're setting up your fitness plan, it's important to assess the larger scheme of things (your mesocyle, or workouts for the month) and smaller plan (the microcycle, which consists of your weekly workouts).

At the beginning of each week, I like to map out a tentative fitness and meal plan. The best way to achieve success is to set up for it, and even if things change, an ideal strategy for busy people is to have an agenda in place.

In order to create the most effective plan for you, a recommended starting point is to explore your **cardio, strength, and flexibility options.** Remember that an efficient fitness routine includes these main components.

Cardio

Alternate cardio intensities. Aim for two to three (max) HIIT sessions each week on nonconsecutive days, alternating with lower-intensity hill or steady-state (moderate intensity) cardio workouts. Some types of cardio to choose:

- HIIT
- HIIT and steady state
- Steady state
- Cardio class (spin, dance, kickboxing)

Strength

Decide how many days you can dedicate to strength training (aim for one to four days) and based on that determine your muscle split, which consists of the muscle groups you'll work each training day. When you strength train, your muscles need time to recover and repair, so avoid strength training the same muscle groups on consecutive days. For example, it's OK to do arms one day and legs the next, but don't work the same muscles two days in a row (that is, doing biceps curls again if you did them yesterday).

Does yoga count as strength training? I don't personally consider yoga as strength training, even though it's a great method to strengthen muscles and promote a full range of motion through flexibility. I don't classify yoga as strength training because there is not a way to impose additional stressors through weight to the exercises, unless you chose to wear ankle or arm weights (and the safety of doing so is debatable at best). You can only challenge yourself weightwise to a certain point, even though you always have options to make the asanas more challenging. Instead, I like to consider yoga as a flexibility exercise and a sanity saver. It centers me, encourages me to breathe and be present, and has taught me strategies and skills that have translated far beyond the yoga mat.

Study up, ladies! Bookmark this section to come back to when you need a refresher, or when you're looking for ways to change up your strength training split. Maybe take this book with you to a coffee shop to study up. I met the Pilot at a certain coffee house with a green logo. You never know where you may find true love!

Time to meet your muscles: Muscle 101 for rookies and a helpful review for those who strength train regularly.

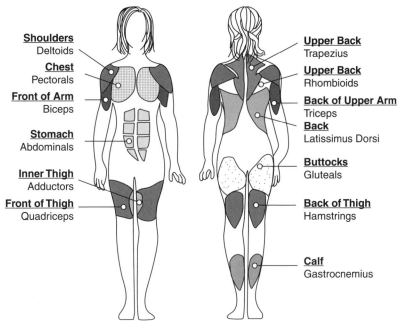

Shoulders
Deltoids

Chest
Pectorals

Front of Arm
Biceps

Stomach
Abdominals

Inner Thigh
Adductors

Front of Thigh
Quadriceps

Upper Back
Trapezius

Upper Back
Rhombioids

Back of Upper Arm
Triceps

Back
Latissimus Dorsi

Buttocks
Gluteals

Back of Thigh
Hamstrings

Calf
Gastrocnemius

Shoulders

Our deltoids comprise three major groups: anterior (front), lateral (middle or side), and posterior (rear). It's important to train all areas of the shoulders to maximize muscular efficiency and reduce the likeliness of shoulder-related injuries. Another critical muscle in the shoulder joint is the rotator cuff, which helps to stabilize the shoulder in everyday activities. Some standard shoulder exercises include the following:*

- Frontal raise (anterior deltoid)

- Lateral raise (lateral deltoid)

- Bent-over fly (rear deltoids)

---

*Descriptions and illustrations of the exercises mentioned in this chapter can be found in Chapter 3. See the exercise index on page 73.

- Overhead press (compound exercise)
- Upright row (compound exercise)

Chest

There are two main components of our pectoral (chest) muscles: pectoralis major and pectoralis minor. Pectoralis major is a larger fan-shaped muscle (located under the breast tissue) and pectoralis minor is a small, triangle-shaped muscle situated beneath the pectoralis major. We use our pectoral muscles often in everyday life, including the muscular exertion to lift a child or a heavy bag of groceries, or engage in arm wrestling (Fitnessista challenges all comers!); they also help keep our arms attached to our body, which is always a good thing. Basic chest exercises include the following:

- Chest press
- Push-up
- Chest fly

Triceps

Our triceps brachii are located on the upper back portion of our arms, and are responsible for extension of the arm from the elbow joint. They're also what many of my clients have referred to as "chicken wings." Please think of a nice name for your triceps. As their name suggests, the triceps have three parts: long head, medial head, and lateral head. As you train your triceps muscles, try to target all three portions. Keeping a close grip will target the triceps more efficiently in cable or barbell exercises. Also, while performing dumbbell triceps exercises, a small rotation at the end of each movement will further fatigue all portions of this muscle group. Basic triceps exercises include the following:

- Triceps dip
- Bent-over triceps extension

- Standing triceps extension

- Triceps press-down (performed using a cable machine at the gym)

Biceps

Our biceps brachii, aka our gun show muscles, are responsible for flexion at the elbow joint. We isometrically stabilize our biceps while carrying heavy items, and they're also a critical component to pick up various items. As the name suggests, there are two parts: the short head and the long head. The classic exercise to work the biceps muscles are regular ol' biceps curls. You can switch these up by performing hammer curls (rotating the weights so the head of the weight is pointing up) or concentration curls at an incline. This creates a longer lever and a more challenging curl variation. Basic biceps exercises include the following:

- Biceps curl

- Hammer curl

- Concentration curl

Abdominals

Ahhhh, the abdominals. The muscles we all want to shred, right? I think it's important to note that six-pack abs are definitely made in the kitchen. You can crunch and plank your little heart out, but if you aren't combining it with clean, whole foods, your efforts may be in vain. The abdominals have a few different components: the transverse abdominals (the deepest portion of our abs, which help to pull our waist in like a corset), the obliques (sides of our abs), and the rectus abdominis. Basic abdominal exercises include the following:

- Plank (transverse abdominis)

- Woodchop (obliques)

- Frog crunch (transverse abdominis)

Back

It's easy to forget that the back is a critical component of our core. You want to make sure to keep a strong back to encourage a balanced core, promoting posture alignment and preventing back ailments. There are two major parts of the back: latissimus dorsi (or lats, the muscles we use to retract our shoulder blades) along with our rhomboids and the erector spinae (extends the vertebral column and is responsible for spinal flexion and extension). Classic back exercises include the following:

- Bent-over row (wide and narrow)

- Deadlift and single-leg deadlift

- Assisted pull-up

- Superman

> What is the core? I like to think of it as your entire body, minus your head and limbs. Glutes and pelvic floor count as core muscles, too!

Glutes

We have three different portions of our gluteus muscles: the minimus (which assists with hip adduction and internal rotation) which is on the outside of our hip, the medius (which assists in external rotation), and the maximus (the booty, which accelerates hip extension). If you stand, point one toe back behind you and try to lift it off the ground, that's all maximus right there. Some favorite classic glute exercises include the following:

- Squat

- Deadlift and single-leg deadlift

- Bridge and single-leg bridge raise

- Hip extension
- Plié squat

Adductor/abductors

Also known as our inner and outer thighs, respectively. These can be a little more challenging to target. Some favorite moves include the following:

- Side leg raises and rotations
- Plié squat with stability ball squeeze (just place a large physioball in between your stance and squeeze on the way up)
- Narrow squats with a small playground ball in between the knees

Quads

The muscles on the front of the thigh, including the vastus medialis, vastus intermedius, vastus lateralis, and rectus femoris. Quads are utilized often in everyday functions, especially in sports and workouts. They're also *super* strong, so don't be afraid to hold some weights. Classic quad exercises include the following:

- Squats and variations
- Lunges and variations

Calves

Calf muscles are not only critical for walking, sprinting, and pointing our toes, but they also take a nice pair of heels over the top. We have two main calf muscle groups: the gastrocnemius (more superficial muscle, closer to the skin) and the soleus (our deeper calf muscle). The most basic way to work your calves includes the following:

- Standing or seated calf raises

Getting your split

As far as strength training goes, there are a few different muscle splits to train.

Synergistic

The muscles that work together to perform a movement. Examples:

- Shoulders/chest/triceps (aka "push muscles")

- Legs (glutes, adductors, abductors, hamstrings, quads, calves) and core

- Back/biceps ("pull muscles")

Antagonistic

Opposing muscle groups to a movement. These would be the muscles used to stop whatever exercise you're doing. Examples:

- Chest/upper back

- Quads/glutes/hamstrings

- Biceps/triceps

- Abdominals/low back

- Shoulders/lats

Lower body and upper body

One day of strength focusing on upper body (shoulders, triceps, biceps, lats, chest) and one lower body + core day (abdominals, low back, hamstrings, glutes, quads, and calves)

Total body circuit

Working through a circuit quickly to exhaust all of the major muscles (shoulders, biceps, chest, triceps, core, glutes/hamstrings, back, quads, and calves). This is one of my favorite techniques because I'm a huge fan of compound movements, which work more than one muscle at once. You're able to move quickly and also be done quickly.

Within your desired method, pick two to three exercises per muscle group. Complete 12 to 15 reps of each exercise, depending on the weight you choose and how much you want to challenge yourself. Ideally, you will want to choose a weight that will make it difficult to complete the last one to two reps.

Sets and reps for your goals

One of the most common questions I'm asked is how many sets and reps to do of each exercise. This is largely dependent on your goals. If you're just getting started in a fitness routine, you'll work slowly through each set and start by performing one set of 10 repetitions for each exercise. From here, you can add in reps (up to 20) and sets (up to 3).

A common goal for intermediate to advanced exercisers is muscular hypertrophy (building lean muscle) and power. Here are some different repetition and set guidelines for each type of goal, whether you're looking to increase muscular endurance, build lean muscle, or increase power.

Reps

One full movement of a single exercise. If an exercise contains multiple parts, performing each portion of the movement will count as one rep.

Sets

Group of consecutive repetitions.

Training intensity

An individual's level of effort, compared with his or her maximal effort, which is usually expressed as a percentage. One RM equals one rep maximum. This is the heaviest weight you could use to "max out" at one full rep. Usually it's smart to get a ballpark idea of this, and with the help of a qualified trainer, determine your personal one rep max.

Training in an unstable environment also increases the training intensity because it requires greater motor unit recruitment, leading to greater energy expenditure per exercise.

Rest interval

The time taken to recuperate between sets. Rest has a dramatic impact on the results of your personal training program. Remember that rest is just as important as work!

Sets and Reps for Your Goals				
	Muscular Endurance and Stabilization	Muscular Hypertrophy	Maximal Strength	Increased Power
Reps	12–20 reps	6–12 reps	1–5 reps	1–10 reps
Sets	1–3 sets	3–5 sets	4–6 sets	3–6 sets
Training Intensity	50%–70% 1 RM	75%–85% 1 RM	85%–100% 1 RM	30%–45% 1 RM
Rest Interval	0–90 seconds	0–60 seconds	3–5 minutes	3–5 minutes

Tempo

If you want to get fancy and focus on the tempo of your exercises, remember that you'll work slowly for muscular endurance and stabilization, moderately for hypertrophy, and quickly for power. Here is an easy way to remember it: If you're working on balance and stabilization exercises, you'll be slowly training to balance through each one. An example of this would be any movement you do standing on one leg or on a challenging surface, such as a BOSU balance trainer. The "power" exercises (all of the cardio exercises in Chapter 3) are "blasts" of effort and activity: quick! I find tempo to be more of an intuitive thing (in other words, don't stress too much about it), but if you're looking for an easy way to change up your strength training routine, tempo is a simple way to do that.

Setting up your weekly strength training plan

Here are some options depending on how much time you can dedicate to strength training each week.

Weekly Strength Training Plans	
1 Day of Strength Each Week	Total body circuit No cardio on this day, strength only
2 Days of Strength Each Week	Option 1: 1 day lower body 1 day upper body Option 2: Total body circuits (make sure these are on non-consecutive days
3 Days of Strength Each Week	Option 1: 1 day lower body 1 day upper body 1 day total body circuit Option 2: Total body circuits (all 3 days nonconsecutive)

(continued)

Weekly Strength Training Plans (*continued*)	
	Option 3: 1 day push muscles (shoulder, chest, triceps) 1 day pull muscles (back and biceps) 1 day legs and core
4 Days of Strength Training Each Week	Option 1: Total body circuits (all 4 days nonconsecutive) Option 2: 2 days upper body 2 days lower body Option 3: 1 day push muscles 1 day pull muscles 2 days total body circuit (nonconsecutive) Option 4: 1 day chest and shoulders 1 day back and triceps 1 day hamstrings, glutes, and quads 1 day back and abs

Flexibility

Be sure to include at least one flexibility option in your regular routine, whether it's a stretching session, yoga class, Pilates, or something else you enjoy. By keeping our muscles flexible, we're able to maintain a full range of motion in our joints and avoid compensation and thus injury. Another key factor to avoiding injury is to keep our muscles *strong* to perform functional movements in exercise and in life. If a muscle is weak, it will cause another muscle to kick in to fill the gap, which can create imbalances and the dreaded injury cycle. Stay strong and flexible!

Stretching before and after workouts

Here's a shocker for you: it's probably not totally necessary. Research is mixed on stretching, and the most recent research indicates that active and static stretching (pre- and postworkout) may not be as beneficial as we once believed. I've always been a huge advocate of stretching, not only because I feel that muscle soreness is reduced postworkout, but I appreciate the Zen and centeredness it provides. I enjoy stretching, so even after learning that it may not be necessary, I'll continue to do it. However, if you don't like stretching before or after your workouts, this is good news for you: you don't have to.

To get the most out of any workout:

- **EXHALE on the EXERTION.** "E" and "E" is how I remember it. You'll always want to exhale on the more challenging part of the movement.

- **Mind to muscle.** Focus on the muscles you're using, whether you're lifting weights or blasting through cardio.

- **Squeeze your booty and keep a tight core.** This is the gold star for getting the most out of any workout.

- **Aim for full range of motion.** When you're completing the full movement of an exercise, the muscle has to work harder for each repetition and thus breaks down more tissue in the process. (This sounds frightening but muscle breakdown encourages repair, rebuilding, and growing back stronger.)

- If you did it yesterday, don't do it today!

Sample weekly fitness plans

The fitness plans below include example exercises and sets to follow. To follow the fitness plans, perform each exercise in a circuit or superset to complete one round. Try to move quickly between exercises with little to no rest between sets. Complete the suggested number of rounds in each circuit before moving on to the next portion of the workout. In the workouts, I've put strength training before cardio, but feel free to switch it up.

To switch things up, substitute different exercises from the same type of workout. For example, substitute the exercises in the upper body workout listed with different upper body exercises of your choice or another of my upper body workouts. The same thing goes for any set strength or cardio option. Mix and match to keep things exciting and also to prevent adaptation from occurring!

Remember to change your routine every four to six weeks!

OPTION 1

Three days of cardio

Two days of strength with upper/lower split

One day of flexibility

SUNDAY
Off

MONDAY
HIIT 1:1 ratio

WARM UP	
Moderate Cardio	5 minutes
HIIT	
15–20 minutes	
30 seconds–1 minute HARD	
30 seconds–1 minute recovery	
COOL DOWN	

TUESDAY

Upper body + steady state

WARM UP	
Moderate Cardio	5 minutes
UPPER BODY BLITZ CIRCUIT	
3 rounds	
Lateral Raise to Biceps Curls	12 reps
Triceps Dips with Pulses	12 full dips and 8 pulses
Renegade Rows	12 reps
Push-ups	12 reps
STEADY STATE	
Moderate Cardio	10 minutes
COOL DOWN	

WEDNESDAY

Off

THURSDAY

Lower body + core

WARM UP	
Moderate Cardio	5 minutes
LOWER BODY SUPERSET 1	
3 rounds	
Squats	10 reps (hold each squat for 10 seconds)
Squat Jumps	30 seconds

(continued)

LOWER BODY SUPERSET 2	
3 rounds	
Lunges	10 reps
Jumping Lunges	30 seconds
LOWER BODY CIRCUIT 3	
3 rounds	
Diamond Bootys	10 full dips and 10 pulses
Plank with Cross and Taps	10 reps on each side
Lateral Lunge to Basketball Throws	10 reps
BONUS	
Weighted Squats	Do as many reps as possible
COOL DOWN	

FRIDAY

Flexibility

Take a yoga class that you love, enjoy a long stretch, or try some Pilates. Make an effort to be more active during the day.

SATURDAY

HIIT 1:1 ratio

Use a different mode of HIIT than the one you used on Monday. If you did the treadmill, try rowing or a jump rope instead. You can also do bodyweight moves, like plyometrics or any of the cardio moves described in Chapter 3 for the hard part of each interval.

WARM UP	
Moderate Cardio	5 minutes
HIIT	
15–20 minutes	
30 seconds – 1 minute HARD	
30 seconds – 1 minute recovery	
COOL DOWN	

OPTION 2

Three days of cardio

Two days of strength with total body circuit

One day of flexibility

SUNDAY

Off

MONDAY

HIIT 2:1 ratio

WARM UP	
Moderate Cardio	5 minutes
HIIT	
15–20 minutes	
1 minute HARD	
30 seconds recovery	
OR	
30 seconds HARD	
15 seconds recovery	
COOL DOWN	

TUESDAY

Total body circuit + steady state

WARM UP	
Moderate Cardio	5 minutes
TOTAL BODY CIRCUIT 1	
2–3 rounds	
Lunges with Weights	10 reps on each side
Squats and Biceps Curls	15 reps
Hold Squats for Upright Rows	15 reps
TOTAL BODY CIRCUIT 2	
2–3 rounds	
Renegade Rows	12
Push-ups	12
Single-leg Bridges	12
STEADY STATE	
Moderate Cardio	10 minutes Keep a slightly uncomfortable quick pace. It's only 10 minutes—you can do it!
COOL DOWN	

WEDNESDAY

Off

THURSDAY

Total body circuit + blitz

WARM UP	
Moderate Cardio	5 minutes
TOTAL BODY CIRCUIT	
15 minutes Do as many rounds as possible	
Burpees	15 reps
Squats	25 reps
Push-ups	10 reps
Bent-over Rows OR Assisted Pull-ups	12 reps
V-ups	15 reps
BLITZ	
10 minutes For each exercise, do as many reps as possible within 1 minute	
Biceps Curls	
Jumping Lunge and Kicks	
Overhead Presses	
Side Crunches	
Planks	

(continued)

BLITZ (continued)	
Side Crunches (opposite side)	
Hammer Curls	
Triceps Dips	
Squats	
Squat Jumps	
COOL DOWN	

FRIDAY

Flexibility

Take a yoga class that you love, enjoy a long stretch, or try some Pilates. Make an effort to be more active during the day.

SATURDAY

HIIT 2:1 ratio + steady state

WARM UP	
Moderate Cardio	5 minutes
HIIT 2-1 ratio	
15–20 minutes	
40 seconds HARD	
20 seconds recovery	
For each exercise, do as many reps as possible within 1 minute	
Burpees	
Lateral Lunge to Basketball Throws	
Squat Jumps with Rotation	

Lateral Lunge to Basketball Throws (opposite side)	
Side to Side Hops	
Squat Jumps (touch the floor)	
High Knees	
Plank Walks and Plank Jacks (moving side to side)	3 plank walks and 5 plank jacks
Mountain Climb and Rolls	
Push-ups	
Vertical Jumps	
Lateral Lunge to Basketball Throws	
Squats	
Tuck Jumps	
Lateral Lunge to Basketball Throws (opposite side)	
STEADY STATE	
Easy Cardio	15 minutes
COOL DOWN	

OPTION 3

Four days of cardio

Two days of strength with upper/lower body split

One day of flexibility

SUNDAY

Off

MONDAY

HIIT 2:1 ratio (distance based)

WARM UP	
Moderate Cardio	5 minutes
HIIT	
15–25 minutes	
0.50 mile HARD	
0.25 mile recovery	
COOL DOWN	

TUESDAY

Upper body + steady state

WARM UP	
Moderate Cardio	5 minutes
	For the first minute, jog in place
	Squat for the second minute
	Jog in place for the third minute
	Squat for the fourth minute
	High knees for the fifth minute
UPPER BODY CIRCUIT	
3 rounds	
For each exercise and each round, do as many reps as possible within 1 minute	

Upright Rows	
Single-leg Deadlifts	
Push-ups	
Triceps Dips	
STEADY STATE	
Moderate Cardio	12 minutes
COOL DOWN	

WEDNESDAY

Off

THURSDAY

Lower body + HIIT

WARM UP	
Moderate Cardio	5 minutes
LOWER BODY SUPERSET 1	
2–3 rounds	
Squats	15 reps
Squat Jumps	30 seconds
LOWER BODY SUPERSET 2	
2–3 rounds	
Lunges	10 reps
Jumping Lunge and Kicks	30 seconds

(continued)

LOWER BODY SUPERSET 3	
2–3 rounds	
Warrior 3 to Half-Moons	10 reps
Single-leg Deadlifts	10 reps
LOWER BODY SUPERSET 4	
2–3 rounds	
Warrior 3 to Half-Moons (opposite side)	10 reps
Single-leg Deadlifts (opposite side)	10 reps
HIIT	
10 minutes	
40 seconds HARD	
20 seconds recovery	
For each exercise, do as many reps as possible within 1 minute	
Side Lunges (switching)	
Wild Burpees	
High Knees	
Knee to Elbows and Push-ups	5 knee-to-elbows on each side and 5 push-ups
Squat Jumps and High Knees back	
Plank Walks and Plank Jacks	5 plank walks in each direction and 5 plank jacks back and forth
Air Jacks	

Tuck Jumps	
Mountain Climbers	
Burpees	
COOL DOWN	

FRIDAY

Flexibility

Take a yoga class that you love, enjoy a long stretch, or try some Pilates. Make an effort to be more active during the day.

SATURDAY

HIIT 1:1 ratio OR steady state

Wild card! This is your choice, depending on how much time you have.

Here are some suggestions:

- Take a favorite cardio or dance class

- Go for a 30 minute easy run

- Do a 20 to 25 minute HIIT workout using any of the methods we've discussed (see page 16 for a reminder)

OPTION 4

Four days of cardio

Two days of strength with total body circuit

One day of flexibility

SUNDAY

Off

MONDAY

HIIT 1:1 ratio

WARM UP	
Moderate Cardio	5 minutes
HIIT	
15–25 minutes	
30 seconds–1 minute HARD	
30 seconds–1 minute recovery	
To switch things up, change the work portion each time, always matching it with your rest recovery	
COOL DOWN	

TUESDAY

Total body circuit + steady state

WARM UP	
Moderate Cardio	5 minutes
TOTAL BODY CIRCUIT 1	
2–3 rounds	
Upright Rows	12 reps
Squats	15 reps
Single-leg Deadlifts	10 reps on each side
Kettlebell or Dumbbell Swings	15 reps

TOTAL BODY CIRCUIT 2	
2–3 rounds	
Assisted Pull-ups or Bent-over Rows	12 reps
Push-ups	10 reps
Walking Lunges	10 reps on each side
STEADY STATE	
Moderate Cardio	10 minutes
COOL DOWN	

WEDNESDAY
Off

THURSDAY
Total body circuit + HIIT

WARM UP	
Moderate Cardio	5 minutes
TOTAL BODY CIRCUIT	
2–3 rounds	
Lateral Lunge to Balance and Overhead Presses	10 reps on each side
Weighted Squats to Biceps Curls	15 reps
Bent-over Rows to Triceps Kickbacks	10 reps
Push-up to Side Planks with Knee Tucks	10 reps on each side

(continued)

HIIT	
8 Tabata rounds*	
30 seconds – 1 minute recovery between each round	
1 Tabata round =	
20 seconds HARD	
10 seconds recovery	
Do as many reps of each exercise as possible within 30 seconds	
Perform this set twice for a total of 8 Tabata rounds	
High Knees	
Burpees	
Mountain Climbers	
Squat Jumps with Rotation	
COOL DOWN	

FRIDAY

Flexibility

Take a yoga class that you love, enjoy a long stretch, or try some Pilates. Make an effort to be more active during the day.

SATURDAY

HIIT 1:1 ratio OR steady state

Wild card! This is your choice, depending on how much time you have.

Here are some suggestions:

- Take a favorite cardio or dance class
- Go for a 30 minute easy run

*These are INTENSE. If you need to reduce the amount or modify, be sure to do so. Always listen to your body. It should feel extremely challenging but never unimaginable or painful.

- Do a 20 to 25 minute HIIT workout using any of the methods we've discussed

OPTION 5

Five days of cardio

Two days of strength with upper/lower split

One day of flexibility

SUNDAY

Off

MONDAY

HIIT 1:1 ratio

WARM UP	
Moderate Cardio	5 minutes
JUMP ROPE HIIT	
20 minutes	
15 seconds HARD	
15 seconds recovery	
40 rounds	
It will go by quickly, I promise!	
Note: To change things up, try doing cross country–style jumps, high knees, or even some double unders. If you don't have a jump rope, no worries, try high knees or another cardio move you "love" that will elevate your heart rate within the 15-second set	
COOL DOWN	

TUESDAY

Upper body blitz + steady state

WARM UP	
Moderate Cardio	5 minutes
UPPER BODY BLITZ SUPERSET 1	
3 rounds	
Biceps Curls	12 reps
Triceps Dips	12 reps
Push-ups	Complete as many as possible in 1 minute
UPPER BODY SUPERSET 2	
3 rounds	
Chest Presses	12 reps
Bent-over Wide Rows	12 reps
Assisted Pull-ups	Complete as many as possible in 1 minute
UPPER BODY SUPERSET 3	
3 rounds	
Upright Rows	12 reps
Single-leg Deadlifts	12 reps

STEADY STATE	
Easy Cardio	10–20 minutes
	Adjust the length of this portion of your workout depending on how long the strength portion takes
COOL DOWN	

WEDNESDAY
Off

THURSDAY
Lower body

WARM UP	
Moderate Cardio	5 minutes
LOWER BODY CIRCUIT	
2–3 rounds	
Squats	15 reps
Squat Jumps	45 seconds
Walking Lunges	10 reps on each side
Jumping Lunges	45 seconds
Bench Diamond Bootys and Pulses	15 reps of each
COOL DOWN	

FRIDAY
Flexibility

Take a yoga class that you love, enjoy a long stretch, or try some Pilates. Make an effort to be more active during the day.

SATURDAY
HIIT 2:1 ratio

WARM UP	
Moderate Cardio	5 minutes
HIIT the Floor! Workout	
20 minutes 40 seconds HARD 20 seconds recovery 20 rounds	
Squat Jumps with Floor Touches	5 reps
Lateral Lunge to Basketball Throws (alternating legs)	5 reps
Burpees	5 reps
Plank Walks with Plank Jacks	5 reps
COOL DOWN	

OPTION 6

Five days of cardio

Three days of strength with total body circuit

One day of flexibility

SUNDAY
Off

MONDAY

Total body circuit + HIIT

WARM UP	
Moderate Cardio	5 minutes
TOTAL BODY CIRCUIT	
2–3 rounds	
Reverse Lunges to Squats	12 reps on each side
Single-leg Deadlifts and Biceps Curl to Overhead Presses	12 reps
Triceps Dips (Challenge: Straight Legs or Weighted)	15 reps
HIIT BLITZ	
5 minutes or 2–3 rounds 40 seconds HARD 20 seconds recovery For each exercise, do as many reps as possible within 1 minute	
High Knees	
Jumping Lunges	
Squat Jumps with Rotation	
Burpees	
Donkey Hop to One Leg Reaches	
COOL DOWN	

TUESDAY

Flexibility

Take a yoga class that you love, enjoy a long stretch, or try some Pilates. Make an effort to be more active during the day.

WEDNESDAY

Moderate steady state

Warm up and complete 30 minutes of moderate steady state. Do anything you enjoy!

Here are some suggestions:

- Take a favorite cardio or dance class

- Go for an easy 30 minute run

THURSDAY

Total body circuit + HIIT

WARM UP	
Moderate Cardio	5 minutes
TOTAL BODY CIRCUIT	
10 minutes	
Do as many rounds as possible	
Squats	15 reps
Upright Rows	15 reps
V-ups	15 reps
Elevated Push-ups	15 reps
Lunges with Rotation	10 reps on each side

Sprinting HIIT
10 minutes
0.25 mile HARD
0.25 mile recovery
COOL DOWN

FRIDAY

Easy steady state

Warm up and complete 30 minutes of easy, recovery steady state. Do anything you enjoy!

Here are some suggestions:

- Take a leisurely hike
- Take a dance class
- Go spinning

SATURDAY

Total body circuit + HIIT 2:1 ratio (repeat the same circuit and HIIT from Monday)

WARM UP	
Moderate Cardio	5 minutes
TOTAL BODY CIRCUIT	
2–3 rounds	
Reverse Lunges to Squats	12 reps on each side
Single-leg Deadlifts and Biceps Curl to Overhead Presses	12 reps
Triceps Dips (Challenge: Straight Legs or Weighted)	15 reps

(continued)

HIIT Blitz	
5 minutes or 2–3 rounds	
40 seconds HARD	
20 seconds recovery	
For each exercise, do as many reps as possible within 1 minute	
High Knees	
Jumping Lunges	
Squat Jumps with Rotation	
Burpees	
Donkey Hop to One Leg Reaches	
COOL DOWN	

OPTION 7

Five days of cardio

Three days of strength with push/pull splits

One day of flexibility

SUNDAY

Off

MONDAY

Upper body + HIIT

WARM UP	
Moderate Cardio	5 minutes
UPPER BODY CIRCUIT 1	
3 rounds	
Upright Rows	12 reps

Push-up	12 reps
Chest Presses	12 reps
UPPER BODY CIRCUIT 2	
3 rounds	
Overhead Presses	12 reps
Push-ups to Side Planks	12 reps
Chest Flys	12 reps
HIIT	
15 minutes	
0.25 mile HARD	
0.25 mile recovery	
COOL DOWN	

TUESDAY

Flexibility

Take a yoga class that you love, enjoy a long stretch, make a date with the foam roller, or try some Pilates. Make an effort to be more active during the day.

WEDNESDAY

Moderate steady state

Warm up and complete 30 minutes of moderate steady state. Do anything you enjoy!

Here are some suggestions:

- Take a favorite cardio or dance class
- Go for an easy 30 minute run

🍃 *THURSDAY*

Lower body and core + HIIT

WARM UP	
Moderate Cardio	5 minutes
LOWER BODY AND CORE CIRCUIT 1	
3 rounds	
Curtsy Lunges	10 reps on each side
Squat Jumps with Rotation	30 seconds
Warrior 3 to Half-Moons	10 reps on each side
LOWER BODY AND CORE CIRCUIT 2	
3 rounds	
Plié Squats	12 reps
Plié Squats with Jumps	12 reps
Circle Abs	10 reps on each direction
Single-leg Bridges	10 reps on each side
HIIT	
10 minutes	
40 seconds HARD	
20 seconds recovery	
For each exercise, do as many reps as possible within 1 minute	
Jumping Lunge and Kicks (alternate legs)	
Squat Kicks	
Side-to-side Hops	

Donkey Hop to One-leg Reaches	
Mountain Climb and Rolls	
Plank Hops	
Burpees	
High Knees	
Squat Jumps	
Squat Jumps or Tuck Jumps	
COOL DOWN	

FRIDAY

Easy steady state

Warm up and complete 30 minutes of easy, recovery steady state. Do anything you enjoy!

Here are some suggestions:

- Take a leisurely hike
- Take a dance class
- Go spinning

SATURDAY

Back and biceps + HIIT

WARM UP	
Moderate Cardio	5 minutes
BACK AND BICEPS BURNER CIRCUIT	
3 rounds	
Biceps Curls	12 reps

(continued)

BACK AND BICEPS BURNER CIRCUIT (*continued*)	
Renegade Rows	10 reps
Single-leg Rows	10 reps, alternating legs
Hammer Curls	10 reps
HIIT	
Any ratio or distance-based HIIT of choice	15–25 minutes
COOL DOWN	

OPTION 8

Five days of cardio

Three days of strength with upper/lower split

One day of flexibility

SUNDAY

Off

MONDAY

Upper body + HIIT

WARM UP	
Moderate Cardio	5 minutes
UPPER BODY CIRCUIT	
3 rounds	
Bent-over Rows	12 reps
Triceps Extensions	12 reps
Upright Rows	12 reps
Chest Flys	12 reps
Push-ups	30 seconds

HIIT
20 minutes
0:00 – 10:00 alternate between 0.10 mile HARD, 0.10 mile recovery
10:00 – 20:00 alternate between 0.25 mile HARD, 0.25 mile recovery
COOL DOWN

TUESDAY

Flexibility

Take a yoga class that you love, enjoy a long stretch, or try some Pilates. Make an effort to be more active during the day.

WEDNESDAY

Moderate steady state

Warm up and complete 30 minutes of moderate steady state. Do anything you enjoy!

Here are some suggestions:

- Take a favorite cardio or dance class

- Go for an easy 30 minute run

THURSDAY

Lower body + HIIT

WARM UP	
Moderate Cardio	5 minutes
LOWER BODY CIRCUIT	
3 rounds	
Lunges	20 reps
Jumping Lunges	30 seconds
Squats	15 reps

(continued)

LOWER BODY CIRCUIT (*continued*)	
Squat Jumps	15 reps
Tuck Jumps	15 reps
Planks with Leg Raises	10 reps on each side
HIIT	
10 minutes 30 seconds HARD 30 seconds recovery Alternate between two high-intensity cardio exercises of your choice. (I'll suggest side-to-side hops and high knees!)	
COOL DOWN	

FRIDAY

Easy steady state

Warm up and complete 30 minutes of easy, recovery steady state. Do anything you enjoy!

Here are some suggestions:

- Take a leisurely hike
- Take a dance class
- Go spinning

SATURDAY

Total body circuit + HIIT

WARM UP	
Moderate Cardio	5 minutes

TOTAL BODY CIRCUIT	
15 minutes	
Do as many rounds as possible	
Burpees	15 reps
Squats	25 reps
Push-ups	10 reps
Bent-over Rows OR Assisted Pull-ups	12 reps
V-ups	15 reps
HIIT	
15–20 minutes	
30 seconds–1 minute HARD	
30 seconds–1 minute recovery	
COOL DOWN	

Creating your monthly workout plan

Create a goal for each month when it comes to your training, as well as a specific muscle group split according to the above options. Maybe one month you're going to do total body circuits three times a week with cardio in there; the next month you'll do an upper/lower body training split. Creating a solid training plan not only makes it easier to remain mindful of your strategy, but also helps to develop a nice flow to your workouts as you aren't scrambling around with a different plan.

Each month, change up your muscle group split. This will keep your body guessing and give you something exciting to look forward to.

Some tips for long-term planning for optimal fat loss include the following:

- Exercise 3 to 10 hours total per week

- Include at least one day of full rest each week

Month 1

- Start with low-intensity cardio

- Focus on stabilization (balance exercises), moving quickly in a circuit. You'll use lighter weights for these exercises, and try to perform exercises standing on one leg or adding a balance challenge (like a Bosu Balance Trainer)

- Slower tempo for reps (at least five seconds), and higher reps (12 to 20 per exercise)

- One to three sets of each exercise

Month 2

- Increase cardio intensity

- Focus on strength building exercises, followed by balance training—you'll start with classic strength exercises (moderate weights) and follow them with balance and/or core work, either through plank combinations or surface changes (Warrior 3 to half-moon is a great exercise to add here)

- Increase the weights that you're using

- Instead of working quickly in a circuit, fatigue each muscle group by completing three sets of each exercise with 30 to 60 seconds of rest in between

Month 3

- Increase cardio intensity

- Focus on power exercises (explosive movements including plyometrics). The cardio exercises in Chapter 3 are all ideal options

- Strength supersets (working opposite muscle groups back-to-back in a circuit)

- Alternate between strength and power exercises (such as a biceps curl followed by a jump squat)

When you don't have a lot of time

So what to do if you don't have more than 10 minutes at a time to work out?

Split it up. Ideally, you'll finish your workout in one set, but if you need to split it up into three 10-minute bouts throughout the day (or night shift!), that's totally fine. A split-up workout trumps a nonexistent one, so don't let the lack of huge time blocks deter you. Remember the excess postexercise oxygen consumption (EPOC) thing? If you work out in small bursts throughout the day, you'll be burning more calories as your body works to bring itself back to a recovery state. More EPOC = more calories burned throughout the day. Also, if you split up your workout, since you've had time to rest there's a chance that you could get in a stronger one for each set.

Find out when you're most energized. If you feel good before heading into work, set your alarm for a few minutes earlier and get in a quick workout. You'll feel a boost of feel-good endorphins, and from my experience, will be more likely to make healthy choices for the day.

Put the distractions away. If you're short on time and want a quick workout, you need to focus and put the reading away. While it's an enjoyable way to pass the time, you're not giving 100% to your workout. Remember, if you work out smarter you don't have to work out longer.

Focus on clean eats. The entire second half of this book consists of nutrition guidelines, recipes, and tips for planning, but it's important to mention now as it has a huge impact on success. It's often said that physical appearance is 80% nutrition, 10% genetics, and 10% exercise. I'm a believer. By eating well, even if you don't have the opportunities to work out as often, you'll still see dramatic results. Of course, workouts have tremendous health benefits, but they aren't the end-all-be-all for physical results. It's actually much easier to lose weight and fat from changes in diet than it is to out-exercise a mediocre diet. So what's the most efficient method? Focus on *both* clean eating and an effective workout routine to speed up your results and create a lifestyle you can easily maintain.

Be patient with yourself. I can't emphasize this enough. Stress and exhaustion are tricky beasts and will encourage your body to hold onto fat. When we become stressed, our body's "flight or fight" response triggers a release of cortisol. When we're stressed, we may tend to turn to eating more than necessary, which can cause weight gain (and that blah feeling following overindulgence). If you're exhausted, rest. Chances are that you wouldn't be able to get an effective workout anyway, and if you rest up, you can make your next gym session even more powerful. Be kind to yourself and listen to your body; it will tell you when it needs a break. Speaking of breaks, it's also important to remember that rest will encourage results from your hard work. Try to avoid the spiral into overtraining, which is especially easy when you're just getting started with a new routine and want to do everything possible to obtain your goals.

> Quality over quantity, always. Ten beautiful and safe squats are better than 100 sloppy ones.

Avoiding overtraining

Overtraining is another "gotcha," especially if you enjoy what you're doing and have no problem logging extra gym time. Here's the problem: if you do too much, it could hurt you in the form of results or even injury. When you're overtraining, you're exhausting the system without providing adequate rest and recovery time. In doing so, it could lead to adrenal fatigue and hormone complications, injury from overuse and also through hypertrophy, when the body feasts on its own muscles, leaving the smooshy stuff behind.

In many cases of overtraining, the body is also burning far more than it consumes. When the body's calorie deficit is too great, the body adapts by lowering the resting metabolic rate (RMR), which means that this will screw up your metabolism. With a lower RMR, all activities will then have a lower calorie burn, including basic everyday activities (also referred to as NEAT: nonactive thermogenesis).

This becomes a cycle that is difficult to break, and if you notice that you're eating too little for your activity level, slowly increase your caloric intake to a safe level. I don't ever recommend going below 1,500 calories per day.

As far as overtraining goes, here are some symptoms:

- Unusually elevated heart rate

- Dreading workouts

- Injury

- Increase in sickness or infections

- Inadequate sleep

- Decrease in performance

- Chronic fatigue

If you start to feel any symptoms from potential overtraining, take some time to evaluate your routine. Include rest days and base the amounts of rest on how you feel following your workouts. For example, if you have an extreme case of delayed onset muscle soreness (DOMS) following a workout, take some time off until you feel better. An Epsom salt bath, massage, date with the foam roller, and icing are all great ways to prevent and decrease muscle soreness.

Working out when you're sick

Many fitness professionals will agree that you can resume your workout if you feel up to it, assuming you do not have a fever and are no longer contagious. If you want to work out on your own while you're sick (that is, you're not putting other participants at risk of sickness with your activity), you can do so if you've checked with your doc. Usually the saying is, if you feel sick above the neck (coughing, sneezing, sore throat, etc.), it's OK to work out; if you feel sick below the neck (body aches, chills, fever), you should rest until you feel better. Usually your body will tell you if you're ready to resume your activity levels. Again, always heed the words of a medical professional.

Some tips:

- **Take your time to warm up**. Assess how you're feeling within the first few minutes of your workout.

- **Decrease the duration.** Try a shorter workout during your first attempt back in the game. If you feel great afterward, you'll know it's OK to increase the time for your next session.

- **Hydrate!** Drink plenty of water before, during, and after your workout.

Fitness gadgets

I truly believe that in order to get an awesome workout all you really need is your own body weight, some comfy sneaks, and some motivation. That being said, there are a variety of ways to gauge and track your fitness habits, as well as some simple tools to assist your workout. Here are a couple that I've found helpful on my own fitness journey:

- **Interval timer.** There are some different interval timers, including some that you can download on your phone for convenience. I prefer the Gymboss models that clip on to your shirt. That way, you aren't stuck lugging your phone around the gym and can set it to the vibrate setting (so fellow gymgoers don't have to hear the beeps signaling the rest and work periods).

- **Heart rate monitor.** While not the most accurate predictor of calorie burn, they're pretty darn close for the price. Heart rate monitors also give ideas of improvements and patterns over time, and can give a little nudge when you could be working harder. Also, if you're following the suggested fitness zones on pages 4 and 5, then you'll know that you're exactly where you need to be for your interval training. You can always go by perceived exertion, but if you're a numbers person like yours truly, some fitness data can be insightful.

- **GPS watch.** This is especially helpful for my runner friends out there. It will tell you your distance, pace, and cheer you along the way. If you're training for a race, a GPS watch can be a fabulous training buddy.

Chapter 3

The Moves: Exercise Index with Form Cues and Photos

Exercise index

Since reading about what to do can be a little confusing, I've included photos and form cues to make these exercises a little easier to understand. You can combine any of these moves into your own workout. They're broken down by category, so any of the moves in one category can be an easy substitution in the example routines as a way to shake things up.

Cardio

Air jacks

For this movement, propel yourself off the floor, performing a traditional "jack" type movement. Beginners: stick to regular jumping jacks, or modified jacks, using one leg out and in at a time.

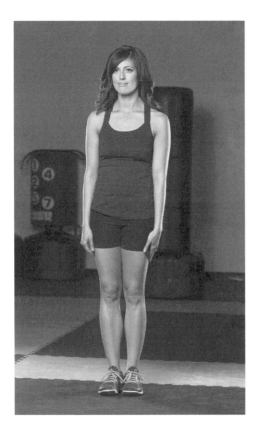
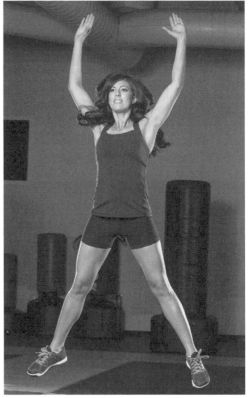

Burpee

Begin with your feet shoulder width apart. Keeping your chest lifted, plank your hands on the floor. Jump (or beginners: walk) your feet back into a classic plank position. Jump or walk your feet back to your hands, and jump up vertically, reaching your hands toward the ceiling. To make this movement even more challenging, add a push-up after jumping back to plank and/or add a tuck jump (exhaling and bending your knees in toward to your stomach) on the vertical jump portion.

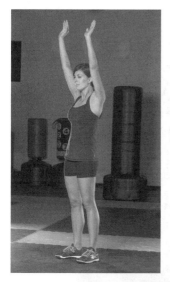
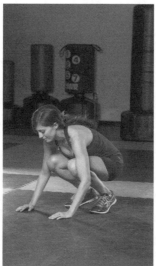
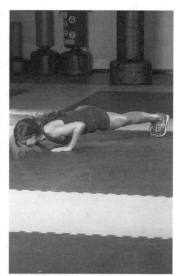

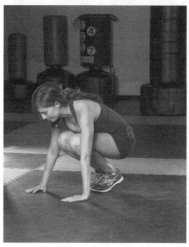
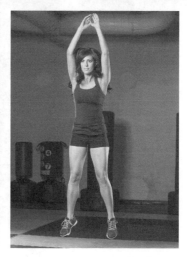

Donkey hop to one-leg reach

Shifting your weight into your hands, use your core to jump and lift both feet off the ground. As you land, kick one leg through and bring the opposite arm to rest on your head. If this is too much, try plank hops, jumping from a plank to bring both feet to the right of your hands (hands remain planted), back to plank, and then jumping to the opposite side.

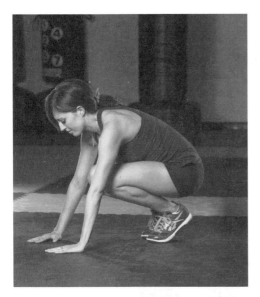
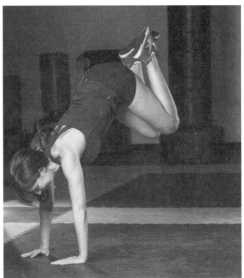
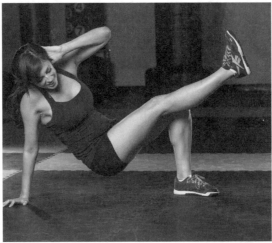

High knees

Use your core to jog in place, lifting each knee up to belly button height. Remember to keep a good posture and take deep breaths. Beginners can march in place, emphasizing core strength and touching each knee with that same hand.

Jumping lunge and kick

Come into a regular lunge position, making sure that your front knee doesn't extend past your toes as you sink down. Keeping your chest lifted and core tight, jump and land in a lunge on the opposite side. Do this three times before lifting your back leg and engaging your core to bring it into a front kick. Beginners: perform regular reverse lunges without jumping.

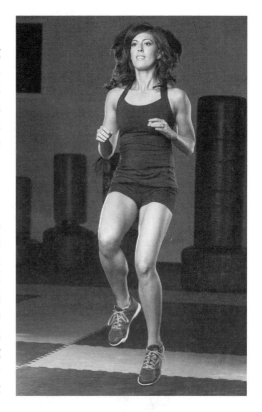

Jump rope

A jump rope is an effective and inexpensive cardio option. You can perform regular jumps—make sure to jump over the rope by alternating feet—or switch things up by doing high knee jumps (bending the knees up toward your core by engaging your abs), cross country jumps (feet stay close to the ground; one foot in front, one slightly behind, and jump to switch), or double unders (one jump for every two full rotations of the jump rope).

Kettlebell or dumbbell swings

It's tempting to think of this exercise as one that's created by your arms, but the power for the movement comes from your legs, booty, and core. Stand with feet a little more than hip distance apart, and hold a dumbbell or kettlebell between your knees. Keep your chest lifted, hold onto that weight for dear life, and carefully start to let it sway forward and backward to gain momentum. When you're ready to start your set, exhale as you swing the weight up to shoulder height, and "snap" your booty forward by using your glutes. Each time you swing up, exhale, and use your legs and core to drive the movement. If you feel as if you need more control, you may need a heavier weight.

Knee to elbow

In a standard plank position, bring your weight forward, rounding the spine and bringing same knee to same elbow. Think about contracting your obliques. To make the movement more challenging, add a plank jack. Come back to plank with a flat back and perform 5 to 10 plank jacks before repeating on the other side. Beginners: instead of doing plank jacks, walk your feet out and together in a plank position, reducing the force of the impact on your wrists.

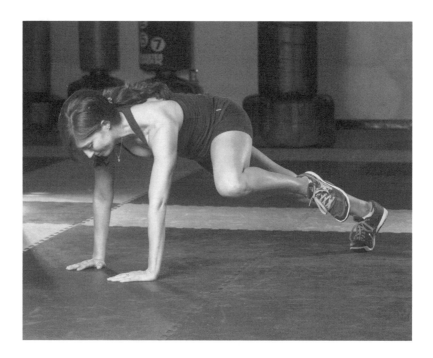

Lateral lunge to basketball throw

Bring one knee into a deep bend, with the toes of that foot pointed out at a 45-degree angle. Keeping the other leg straight, spring up to throw an imaginary basketball. Repeat for the duration of your interval set before switching to the opposite side.

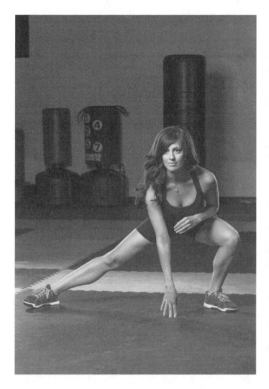 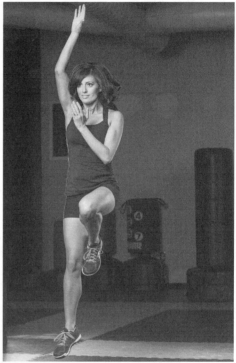

Mountain climbers and roll

Come into a plank position and perform four mountain climbers on each side. Carefully lower yourself to the floor, extend arms overhead, and roll. Push up into a plank position, repeating the mountain climbers, and roll the opposite way. It's kind of a playful—when was the last time you rolled around on the floor?—but killer cardio exercise! Go for it!

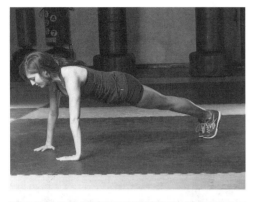

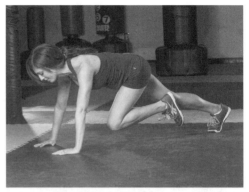

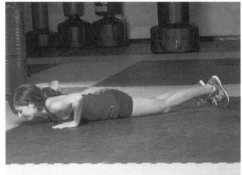

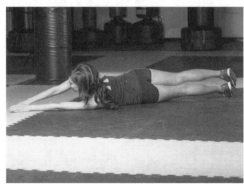

Plank jack to mountain climbers

Keeping your hips low and your spine in a straight line, complete a specified number of plank jacks followed by the same amount of mountain climbers. During the mountain climbers, be sure to use your core and exhale to bring your knees in toward your chest. Beginners: keep this move low impact by "walking" through each movement instead of jumping.

Plank walk to burpee

Start in a standard plank position, with hips low, wrists stacked directly under your shoulders and pressing back through your heels. "Walk" your right arm and right foot out to the right and then bring your left arm and foot to meet it. Complete three before going into a burpee variation of your choice. Walk to the other side and repeat.

Side-to-side hops

Start squatting low, with both palms pressing firmly into the ground. Engage your core and, keeping both feet glued together, hop both feet to the right side of your hands. Take a nice deep inhale, and on your exhale, hop to the left. Repeat back and forth for the duration of the interval set.

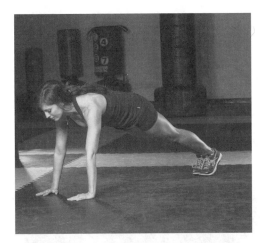
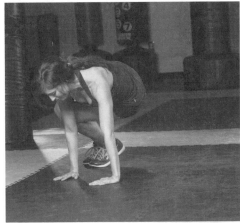
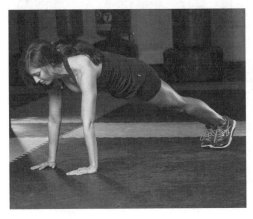
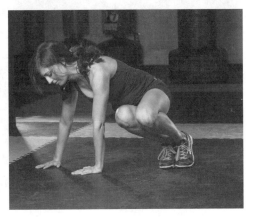

Squat and kick

For this move, sit low into a squat, with legs slightly wider than hip distance. Next, hop one foot toward the center and, using your glutes, kick the other leg out to the side. For your kick, press out through your heel and point your toe straight forward. Come back into your squat and kick again. Repeat for the entire cardio set before alternating to the other side.

Squat jumps

There are quite a few squat jump variations you can do! For the basic movement, come into a deep squat with chest lifted, core tight, and your weight in your heels (booty back). Jump up, reaching your arms up toward the ceiling and land with a soft knee. Squat and repeat. Beginners can avoid jumping by squatting and touching the floor, then reaching up toward the ceiling while rising onto their toes. You can still get the intensity of the movement without the joint impact.

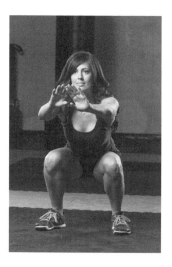
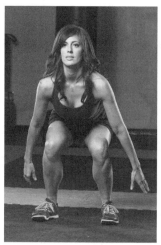
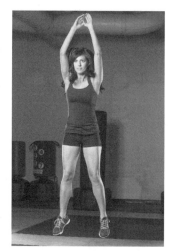

Squat jump with rotation

For the squat jump and rotation, perform your squat facing one side. On the jump, rotate 180 degrees to face the opposite side. This is a fun way to switch up the usual squat jump.

Tuck jumps

For this exercise, jump as high as you can and bring your knees in toward your chest. Make sure to exhale on the jump and use your core to lift your knees. This is a great way to add extra power into a regular burpee. Make sure to land with soft knees.

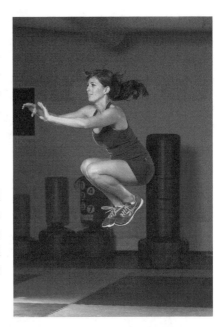

Vertical jumps

Vertical jumps are like squat jumps, minus the squat. You're jumping and reaching toward the ceiling with your hands. Each time you land, be sure to do so with a soft knee. Use your legs to power up, and try to jump a little higher each time.

Wild burpee

This is my favorite burpee variation. Perform the standard squat and touch the floor, jump back into a plank, then do two push-ups. Jump your feet back in, then out to plank, back in, and spring up into a tuck jump. The entire move is eight counts: floor, back, push-up, push-up, in, out, in, JUMP. For the tuck jump, contract your abs, bend your knees, and deep exhale. Land softly. If the tuck jump is too much, a plain vertical jump works nicely.

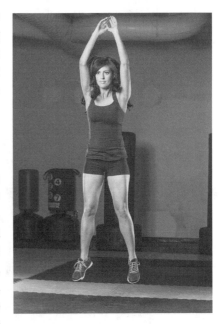

Strength

For strength, there are over a thousand exercises in the sea, but I like to start with the basic functional movements and get fancy from there by adding balance challenges, rotation, holding, pulses, and direction changes. Here are some of the more basic strength training movements as a starting point, and you can build up from these over time to add additional challenge and stressors to keep the body guessing.

Shoulders

Frontal raise

For this exercise, use lighter dumbbells and keep arms at sides—shoulders are relatively small muscle groups and fatigue quickly—and raise the weights in front of you to shoulder height. You can also alternate these with lateral raises.

Lateral raise

For this exercise, use lighter dumbbells and raise the weights out to the sides to shoulder height.

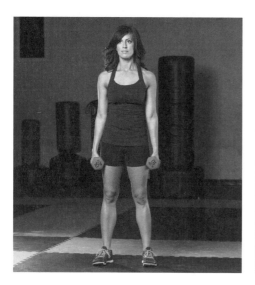 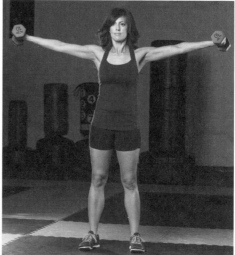

Overhead press

For this exercise, create two 90-degree angles, one with each arm (like a cactus). As you exhale, press the weights up overhead, but avoid clanking the weights together. Come back to your 90-degree angles (not letting the elbows droop below shoulder height to keep some resistance) and press back up.

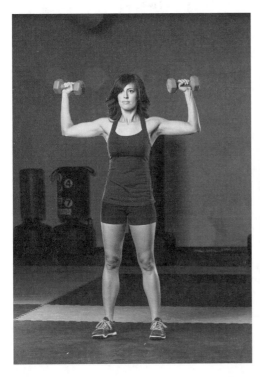 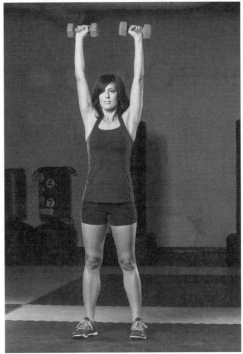

Side-lying lateral raise or plank raise

This is a great way to challenge your core and also make the exercise more challenging without increase the weight. By changing the lever of the workout, it feels much more difficult! You can do this on a bench, resting on a stability ball, or holding onto something sturdy (I've used weight training machines in the past) as you lean and lift.

Upright row

For the upright row, hold moderate weights and lead with your elbows to raise. Keep the weights toward the midline of the body, lower, and repeat.

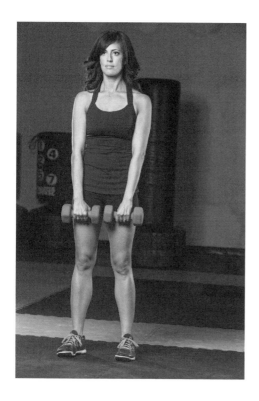 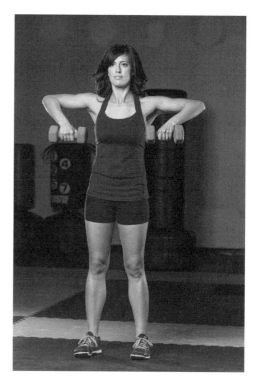

Chest

Chest fly

Lie on your back, knees bent, with feet on the floor about hip width apart. Raise the weights in front of your chest and, keeping a very slight bend in your elbows, open them out to the sides. Keep your arms about shoulder height or slightly lower as you contract your pectoral muscles and bring the weights back to center.

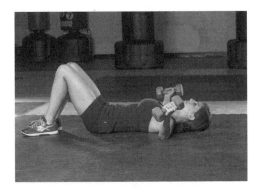 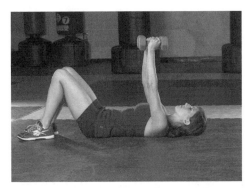

Chest press

The chest press is most easily performed on the floor. Bring your elbows out in line with your shoulders and create a 90-degree angle. Press the weights up in front of you (meeting in front of your chest) and avoid clanking the weights together. As you bring the weights together, focus on engaging the muscles in your chest. (Some women fear strength training their pectoral muscles, as they think it will, um, "shrink the girls." That will not happen; it helps in keeping gravity from taking its toll over time and actually helps to keep everything in place, if you know what I mean....)

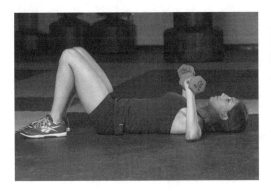 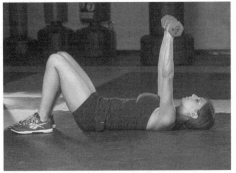

Push-up (variations)

There are a ton of push-up options out there, but remember that the best one is the one that allows you to safely complete a full set. I like to try at least a few clapping push-ups (OK, normal push-ups on my toes) before dropping to my knees for the rest of them. It doesn't matter what type you do; just do them! Keep your spine straight (no hips in the air, and neck in line with your spine instead of dropping forward), hands wide, knuckles pressing into the floor, and exhale on the way up.

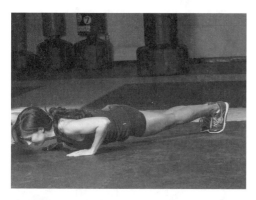
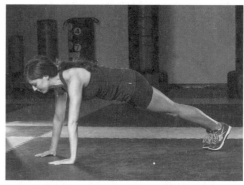
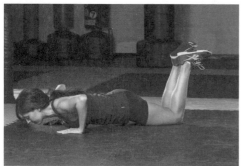
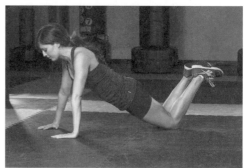

Triceps

Bent-over triceps extension

Hinge forward from your hips, keeping your core tight and a flat back. Bending your elbows, glue your arms to your sides, and then straighten the arms as much as possible. Inhale to bend, exhale to straighten. You can target the various parts of the triceps by rotating from your wrists for palms to face down or up. For this exercise, be sure to maintain a neutral spine and neck position.

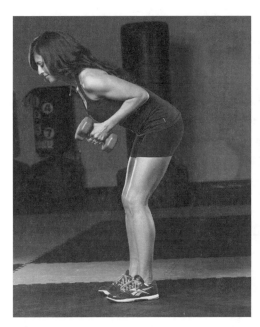 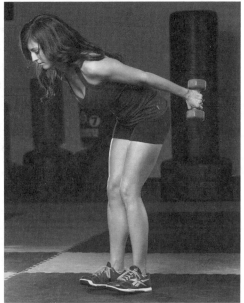

Standing triceps extension

For triceps extensions, be sure to keep your arms framing your head. Avoid letting your elbows shoot out to the sides. Keep the shoulders down and relaxed as you extend the weight up (you can hold one or two weights) and then carefully bend and straighten. For this exercise, core is engaged, feet are hip-width apart, and knees are slightly bent.

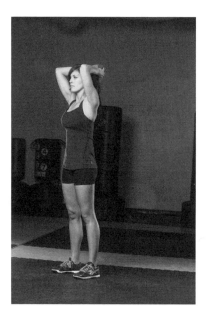 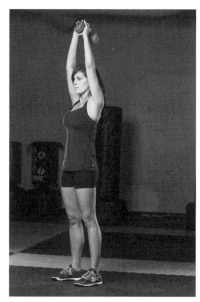

Triceps dips and variations

For triceps dips, point your fingertips toward your toes. You can perform these on a bench (hands on the bench, feet on the floor) or on the floor. As you bend your elbows back, endeavor to keep your hips lifted. Straighten your arms by engaging your triceps. There are quite a few variations you can play with from here. Straight legs is a little more challenging and one leg is even more so. For an extra challenge, place a flat weight on your lap.

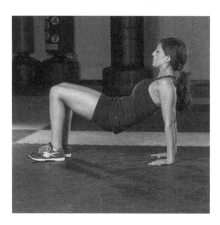 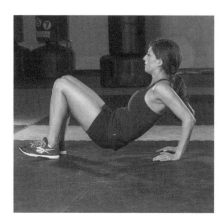

Legs

Calf raise

For this exercise, stand in a neutral position. Lift your heels to come up onto your toes, and carefully lower your heels down about 1 inch above the floor to keep the muscles engaged. Repeat.

Diamond booty

This is one of my all-time favorite glute exercises. Lying on your stomach (prone position), you'll make a diamond with your legs by touching your toes and letting knees fall out to the sides. Place both hands under your forehead and keep a straight spine. Making a small movement, contract your glutes to lift your legs off the floor a few inches. Lower down, without completely resting on the floor. To make this move more challenging, you can perform it on a weight bench (with hips in line with the end of the bench). This will increase the range of motion for the movement and make it more intense. You can also hold a light dumbbell between your feet.

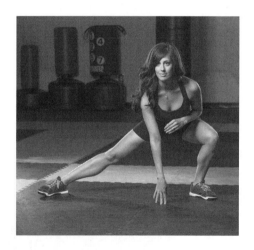

Lateral lunge

To perform the lateral lunge, step one foot far out to the side, letting your heel come to the floor first with the foot angled 45 degrees out. Keeping your other foot on the floor (toes turned slightly in), keep the planted leg straight and bend the other while you sink your hips toward the floor. Make sure to keep your chest lifted. If you're holding dumbbells for a weighted lateral lunge, you can perform a variety of arm strength exercises upon returning to center between each rep, such as a frontal raise.

Lunges and variations (curtsy, tick tock, reverse, walking)

For a basic lunge, your feet should be hip width apart. (I like to say "pretend you're standing on railroad tracks; not a balance beam.") Step as far back with one leg as possible, and lift the back heel off the floor. As you sink down into your lunge, focus on the downward movement instead of moving forward. Chest stays lifted, core stays tight, shoulders are relaxed. Exhale on the way up. Make sure your front knee doesn't shoot forward. There are quite a few fun lunge variations but the basic idea remains the same: sink straight down and squeeze everything to come up.

- Curtsy: Similar to the basic lunge except for the angle of your feet and legs (see images following).

- Tick tock: Perform a forward lunge (stepping one foot forward) and then bring it back to center before completing a lateral lunge with the same leg. Step back to center, then step back to perform a reverse lunge. You will be completing three types of lunges (forward, lateral, and reverse) with one side before switching to the other.

- Reverse: Take a big step back with one foot, keeping feet hip width apart. Lift up through your chest, tighten your core, and sink into a lunge, then step back to center before repeating on the other side.

- Walking: Take a big step forward, and, keeping proper alignment and posture, sink into a lunge. Rise back up to stand and step the opposite foot forward before lunging on the other side, then continue to "walk" and lunge moving forward (for space constraints, take a few walking lunges forward before rotating to lunge back the way you came).

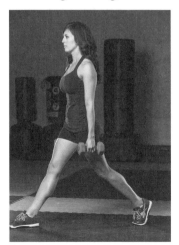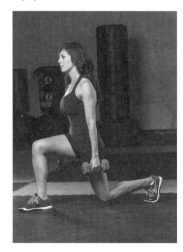

Lunge

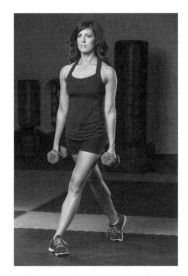
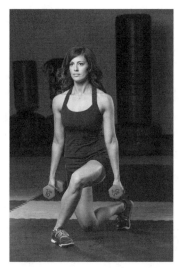

Curtsy lunge

Plié squats

For plié squats, your feet are farther than shoulder distance apart and toes are angled out 45 degrees. Sink down into a squat, keeping your hips in line with your torso (avoid letting your booty shoot back) and knees extending out to the sides. Endeavor to get your thighs parallel to the floor. As you come up from your squat, squeeze every muscle in your legs (inner thighs, outer thighs, glutes, hamstrings, quads, everything).

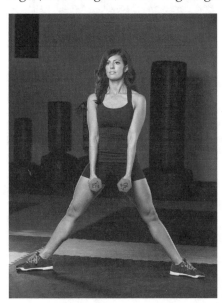
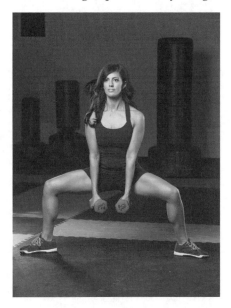

Side leg raises and rotations

To get set up for these exercises, begin on your knees. Lean to one side, and put the bottom hand on the floor in line with your shoulder. Extend your opposite leg out to the side, with your toes pointing straight ahead. For these exercises, focus on stacking your bottom knee and hip joint, as well as your wrist and shoulder. Lift the extended leg up to hip height, and gently lower down. You can also add in small hip rotations moving forward and backward.

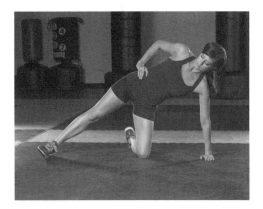 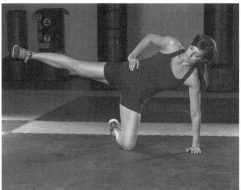

Squat

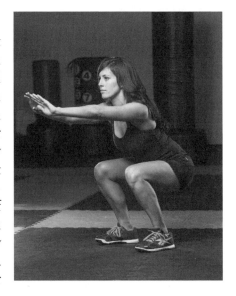

For squats, keep your legs at least hip distance apart and focus on sitting your hips back instead of just down. Chest will remain lifted, core is tight, and exhale on the way up. It is safe to squat your hips low if you have the flexibility and strength in your knees. Just go down as far as you feel comfortable (baby squats are OK if you maintain good form!). Watch your front knees to make sure they don't extend far past your toes. Your weight should be on your heels the entire time.

For weighted squats, just hold a pair of dumbbells or a flat weight against your chest for extra resistance.

Back
Back extension

For this exercise, begin in a prone position, on your stomach. Legs should be extended, and arms should be extended overhead. Contracting your low back (erector spinae), peel your chest off the floor, with arms extended over your head. Endeavor to create length in addition to height, reaching out as well as up. Carefully lower down and repeat. Some variations: lift opposite arms and legs, Pilates swim (raising your torso up and making a faux swimming motion), slightly twist (place arms on the head and as you come up, slightly twist to one side. This is a very small movement; maybe 1 inch to each side).

Bent-over fly

For this exercise, you're targeting your rear delts (the back of your shoulders). Begin in the classic row position: feet hip distance apart, knees slightly bent, hinging forward from your hips, neutral neck, and a flat back. Holding the dumbbells in front of your belly with straight arms, and keeping your arms very slightly bent, raise your arms out to the sides (creating a "T" shape). Lower your back to the start position. Try to keep your arms as straight as possible, but with a tiny bend to avoid locking the joints.

Bent-over row (narrow row, wide row, Is, Ts, and Ws)

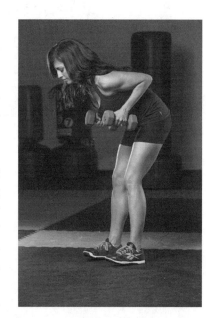

For this exercise, begin with your feet hip width apart, knees slightly bent, and hinge forward from your hips. To perform a narrow row, you'll bring the weights in toward your torso and engage your lats. (Imagine squeezing a lemon between your shoulder blades.) For a wide row, you'll bring your elbows out to the side during the row portion, creating a 90-degree angle (weights perpendicular to your torso). For Is, Ts, and Ws, use lighter weights than you would for your rows, as these exercises target the rear delts, which are a smaller muscle group and fatigue more quickly. Start in the classic row position (hinging forward from your hips, core engaged, and a flat back), and bring the weights up overhead, so you're making an "I" with your body. For the "T," bring the weights out to the sides, in line with your shoulders (same as a reverse fly). For the "W," bend your arms at the elbows, weights pointing up, creating a "W" shape with your arms.

Superman

For this exercise, lie in a prone position (on your stomach) with legs straight and your arms extended forward. Think about tightening your core and, with control, raise your legs and arms off the floor. Your gaze will remain down to keep the spine in alignment. Think about reaching out to create length in addition to lifting off the ground. Carefully lower back down and repeat.

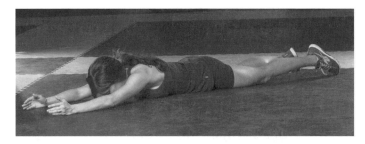

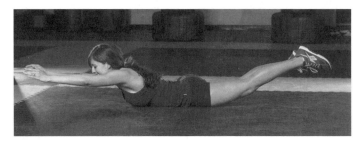

Biceps

Biceps curl

This is the classic biceps exercise. For this one, don't be afraid to lift heavy weights. As I like to tell my clients, your purse probably weighs at least 10 pounds. Start with feet hip distance apart, chest lifted, core tight, and knees slightly bent. Flexing at the elbow, curl the weight in toward your torso before carefully lowering down. Remember to always keep some tension during this movement; avoid letting the weights fall down completely between each rep.

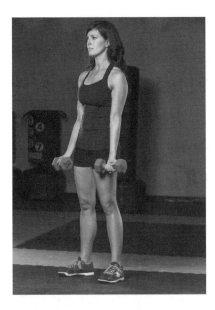 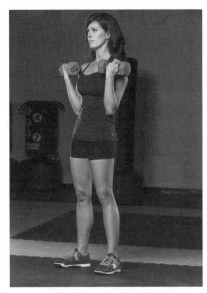

Concentration curl

For the concentration curl, gravity is going to make things a little more exciting. You should perform each curl unilaterally (that is, one side at a time) and change your lever by curling over a slanted weight training bench. Because this puts more pressure on your elbow, you may have to reduce the amount of weight at first. This is an easy variation to make biceps curls more challenging.

Hammer curl

The difference between a regular ol' biceps curl and a hammer curl is that you perform the hammer curl with the weights pointing up (parallel to your torso). This targets the short head of your biceps and is an easy way to change up your routine.

Compound exercises

Compound exercises work more than one muscle group at a time. As you can probably tell, these are my favorite, as they're time-efficient (more muscles in one movement) and also elevate the heart rate. Something to keep in mind for compound exercises: even though there is a lot going on, pay attention to your form. If you need to split the movements up and do each part one at a time until you get the feel for it, I think it's a great idea to become more familiar with the movements. Try them slowly before attempting a full set, and concentrate on the muscles that you're working.

Total body

Bent-over single-leg row

Single leg is just a progression of a regular bent-over row. If you prefer to keep both feet on the floor, no big deal, just make sure they're underneath your hips. For any version of this movement, be sure to keep a flat back, tight core, and squeeze your shoulder blades together during the row.

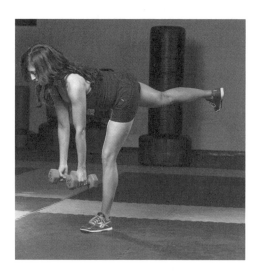 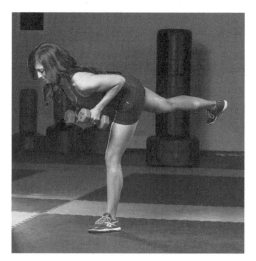

Curtsy lunge and hammer curl

For your curtsy lunge, your front foot is angled 45 degrees out to the side. Step your other back behind and out to the side as much as possible. Sink into a lunge, keeping nice posture and a tight core. As you come up to stand, perform a classic hammer curl with elbows glued to your sides and the head of the weights pointing up.

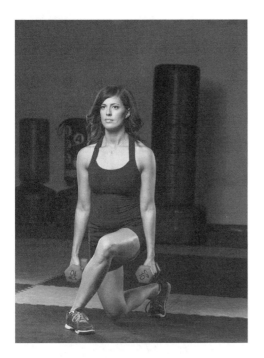
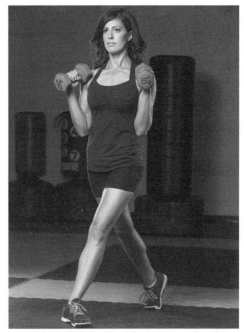

Lateral lunge to balance and overhead press

For this exercise, perform a classic lateral lunge, holding the weights at your sides for extra resistance. As you step your feet back together, remain standing on your stabilizing leg and raise the lunging leg off the floor by bending your knee. Raise the weights up to a 90-degree angle (still balancing on one leg) and perform an overhead press.

Lateral raise to biceps curl

Stand with your feet hip distance apart and perform a classic lateral raise, using dumbbells or resistance bands. Keep a nice tall posture, a slight bend in your elbows, and keep your arms as straight as possible, raising them up to shoulder height. Come back down to start and perform a classic biceps curl, with elbows glued to your sides, bending your elbows, and bringing the weights up toward your shoulders. Lower the weights down again and alternate between the lateral raises and biceps curls to complete the specified number of repetitions.

Lunge and overhead press

During lunges, your stance should be hip width apart. Step one foot back, with your back heel off the ground. Sink into your lunge, making sure to sink downward instead of forward. Watch your front knee to make sure it doesn't extend past your toes. If you perform this movement holding dumbbells, as you stand, you can bring the weights into an overhead press. As you press up, keep your shoulders down and avoid clanking the weights together at the top part of the movement.

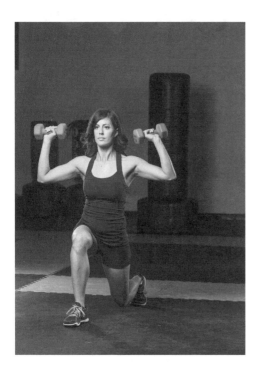 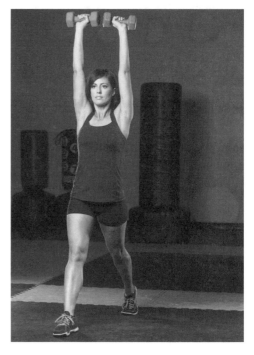

Plié squat to biceps curl or overhead press

During a plié squat, both feet are pointed out at a 45-degree angle, and feet are wide apart (at least shoulder distance). As you squat, aim to have your knees go out over your toes and endeavor to bring your thighs parallel to the ground. Keep your chest lifted and core tight. As you come up to stand, if you're holding weights you can perform a variety of arm strength exercises such as a biceps curl or overhead press.

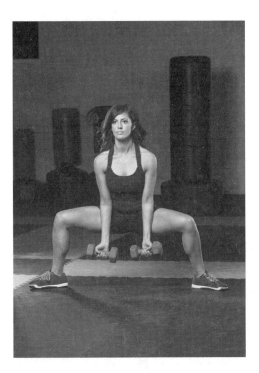 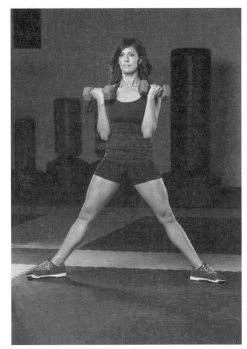

Renegade row

This exercise begins in a basic plank, holding on to a pair of dumbbells. You can also do a modified plank instead, with both knees on the floor and hips in line with your body (no booties in the air!). Make sure that your joints are stacked, with knuckles directly under your shoulders. Engaging your back, bring one weight into a row position, keeping your plank intact. Lower and repeat on the other side.

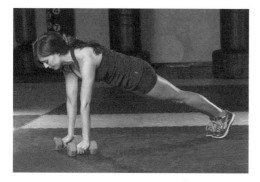
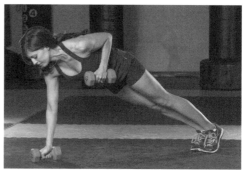

Side plank and lateral raise

This is one of my favorite compound exercises! Come into a side plank (either full or modified by keeping your bottom knee on the floor) and hold a light weight in your free hand. Bring the weight to the center of your core, and keeping your arm very slightly bent, lift it up to shoulder height. Come back to center. For even more of a challenge, you can lift your top leg and touch it to the weight in between each rep.

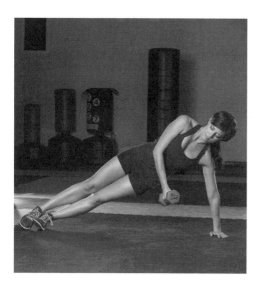
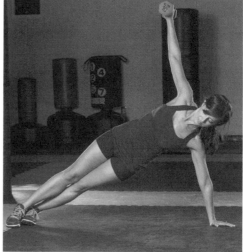

Single-leg deadlift to bent-over row

For a single-leg deadlift, you have a couple of options. Option one is to step one foot behind you, lightly tapping your toes to the floor. Hinge forward from your hips, keeping a tight core and flat back to complete the deadlift. Once you have your balance, you can try option 2: lifting the back leg off the floor. It can come up to hip height as you deadlift, but make sure to keep your hips parallel to the floor. As you rise up from the deadlift, the raised leg can lightly tap the floor before lifting again for each repetition. If a single-leg deadlift is too challenging, experiment with reducing the weight in your back leg until you feel comfortable lifting it off the floor. Keep your back flat by bringing your shoulders back and keeping a tight core. You can perform a wide row, narrow row, or bent-over fly at the end of this movement. Whichever row you decide to do, be sure to keep your hips parallel to the floor.

Squat to single-leg upright row

For this exercise, come into a basic squat with weight in your heels, chest lifted, core tight, and booty back. Watch your knees to make sure they don't extend past your toes. As you rise, come onto one leg (bending and lifting one knee up toward your chest) and perform any arm exercise of choice. For this example, I chose the upright row. Make sure to lead with your elbows for this particular movement.

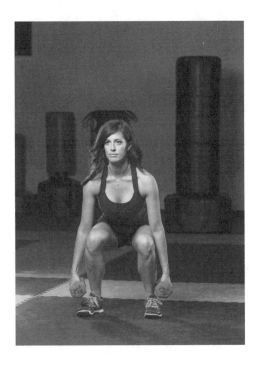 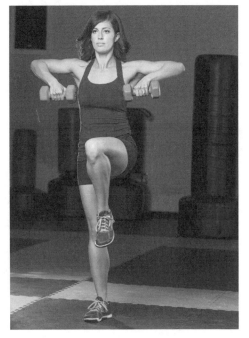

Core/balance
Bridge and single-leg bridge

The bridge, or hip raise, probably ranks high on the slightly inappropriate gym exercise list, but it's a great one. (Unlike the "good girl/bad girl" abduction/adduction machine that is also inappropriate and offers negligible fitness benefits in the bargain.) Make sure to keep your shoulders rooted into the ground and hips even as you lift and lower your hips to the floor. Always keeping resistance, avoid resting the hips on the floor between reps. As an extra challenge, try this with one leg, but keep both knees in the same line.

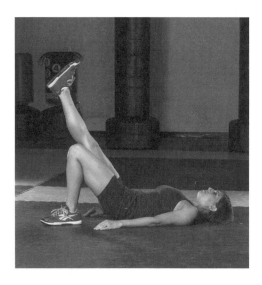 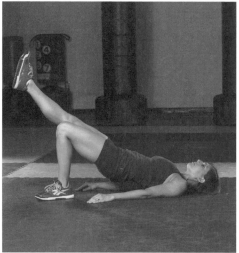

Circle abs

This is a variation of the classic crunch. Point both toes up toward the ceiling and bring your hands into your chest, elbows out. As you exhale, contract your abs and "draw" a circle with your torso. Make 10 circles to one side before repeating in the opposite direction.

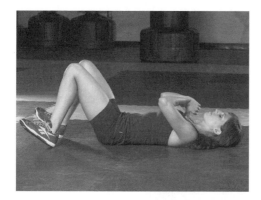
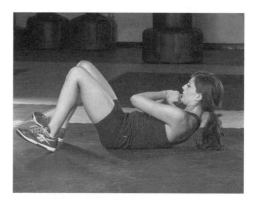

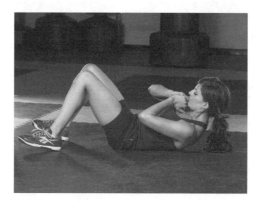

Crunch and side crunch

For your classic crunch, your head should rest in your hands while you lie in a supine position (on your back), knees bent, and feet planted flat on the floor. Engage your abs to carefully lift your head and shoulders off the floor and carefully lower down to repeat. For your side crunch, try to bring one shoulder toward the opposite knee in your crunch position.

Frog crunch

This is one of my favorite core-strengthening moves … just because it's funny looking and works. As a variation of regular ol' crunches, make a diamond shape with your legs (knees out to the sides, toes touching in the middle). As you come up into your crunch, bring your knees toward your elbows. Be sure to exhale on the way up and inhale on the way down.

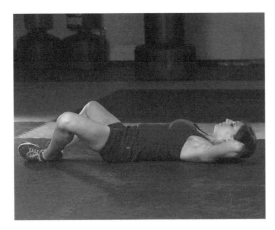 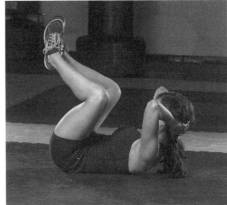

Leg drops

For this exercise, lie supine with your arms either at your side or under your lower back (for more stability). Keep your back pressing into the floor and raise your legs up (so your body is now a 90-degree angle). Slowly lower your legs toward the floor. Maybe you can go 45 degrees, or maybe you can lower to 1 inch off the floor. Exhale and raise your legs back up before repeating. Challenge: hold your legs at the lowest position for three breaths before returning to the start position.

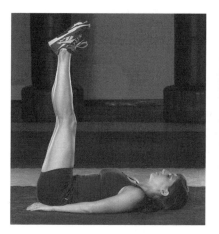
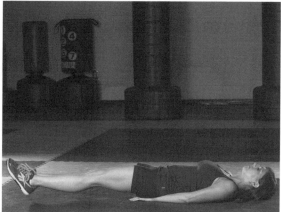

Mountain climbers

Start in a basic plank position, and keeping your hips in line with your body, engage your core and bring one knee in toward your chest. Hop or walk to switch, bringing the opposite knee toward your chest.

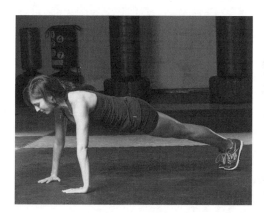
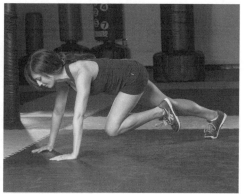

Plank and variations

An ode to the plank. This is one of the most effective and functional total body strengthening exercises. You can start off by keeping your knees on the floor, but hips are down. Be sure that your entire body is in a straight line, with your core engaged and hands or forearms

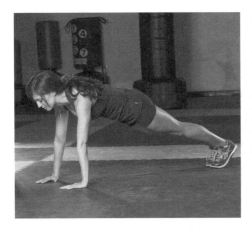

stacked under your shoulders. Some plank ideas: plank jack (add a jumping jack motion with your feet); lift one leg off the ground; saw (sliding forward an inch, back an inch); up and down planks (onto forearms then back onto hands and repeat); hip drops (alternating dropping each hip); the flying plank (both feet and arms off the ground ... just kidding—don't try this at home!).

Jumping plank

For this plank version, keep your hands or forearms planted on the ground and take three tiny jumps, jumping your feet toward your hands. The fourth jump is back to the starting position.

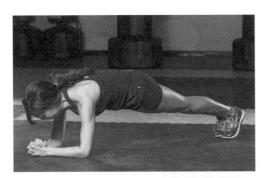 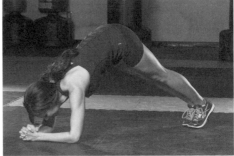

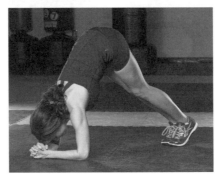

Plank with cross and tap

Come into your classic plank and raise one leg off the ground. Cross it up and over the leg that is still on the floor, and tap it to the ground. Lift and bring it back to the starting position before repeating with the opposite side. This move is easily modified by keeping your knees on the floor and hips down in line with your body.

Push-up to side plank

This is a fantastic total body exercise. Perform a classic push-up (arms at least shoulder distance apart, hands pressing into the floor, and spine straight) before rotating into a side plank. The beauty of this exercise is that it's easily modified (push-up on knees, rotate to side plank, keeping one knee on the floor) and can quickly be made more challenging by keeping one leg off the floor the entire time (one-leg push-up to side plank with the top leg raised).

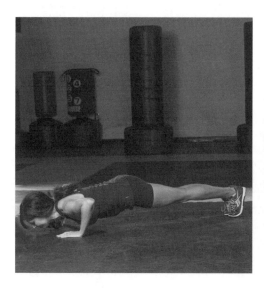
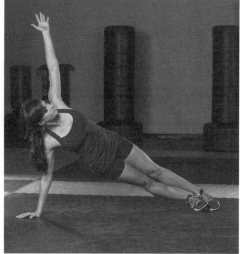

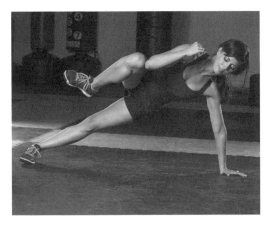

Option: push-up to side plank with knee tuck: add a knee tuck at the top of the movement. Engage your core and bring your top knee in toward your chest before lowering it down slowly with control.

Raised plank and knee tuck

This is a twist on the usual plank, and a great way to add further engagement to your oblique muscles. Elevate your feet by either placing them on a sturdy chair, bench, or the couch, and then using your obliques to alternate bringing each knee in toward your elbow, chest, or opposite elbow.

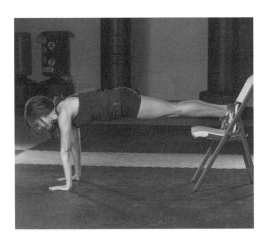
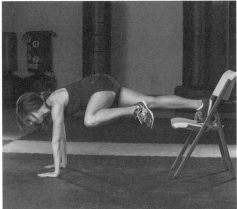

Side plank combo (knee tuck, leg tap)

Just like a traditional plank, there are a ton of *fun* side plank variations to enjoy. You can lift your top leg, perform knee tucks, or use your top arm to lightly tap your thigh.

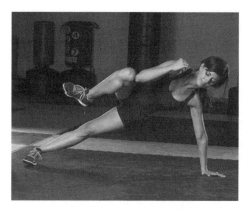

Side plank with knee tuck

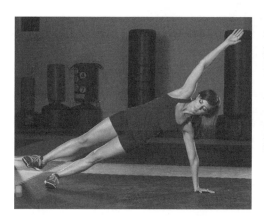

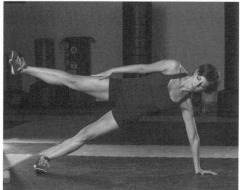

Side plank with leg tap

V-ups and variations

For a traditional V-up, start seated on the floor (or a bench) with fingertips pointing toward your toes. As you exhale, bring your torso up tall and draw one or both knees into your chest. Inhale and bring your torso back as far as possible while extending your legs in front of you. As a challenge, you can perform this move with both legs straight the entire time. To modify, try one leg at a time before attempting both.

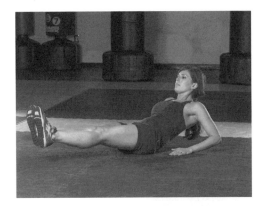
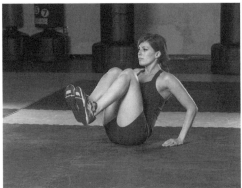
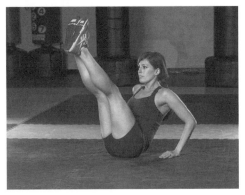

Warrior 3 to half-moon

If you practice yoga, you're already familiar with these movements. As a way to change things up, I love putting them together into a combo, especially between heavy strength sets. It's a fantastic method to simultaneously work your core and balance. For Warrior 3, try to make a capital "T" with your body: arms extended out front, one leg behind you, hips parallel to the floor, and core engaged. Transition by bringing your raised leg and arms in toward your body, and plant one hand to come into half-moon. For the half-moon, your joints are stacked (hand under shoulder, leg under hip bone), and you should focus on creating space by opening your top arm and possibly gazing toward your top arm.

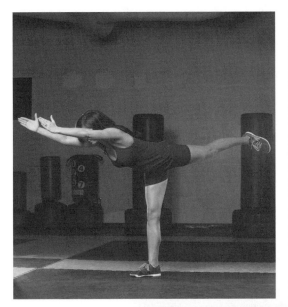
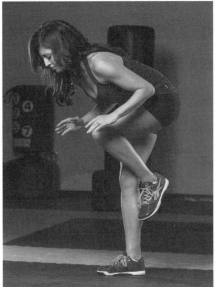
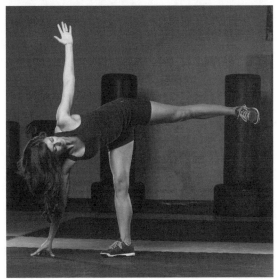

Woodchop

For this exercise, stand either holding a dumbbell or the cable machine, using both hands, up to one side of your body. Rotate your body (making sure to pivot onto the back toes) as you "chop" the weight diagonally down. Return with control back to the starting position.

Chapter 4

Change It Up

Our bodies are intelligent machines. OK, sometimes they make us do silly things (i.e., crowdsurfing—a blast and a hazard on so many levels). But for the most part, they're pretty mind-boggling. The functions that occur throughout the day, including those used to read this book (thank you!!) are pretty astounding. Since our bodies are intelligent machines, they also get bored easily. When you impose the same demands day after day, guess what? They kick it into cruise control. This is also referred to as the SAID principle: specific adaptations to imposed demands.

When I first start training clients, I often find that many of them have been following the same routine yet have been expecting new results. I was also guilty of doing this with my own training in the past. When you don't change your nutrient intake or your fitness activities, your body will give you exactly what you've been giving it: the same exact thing. As I like to say: change creates change. If you alter your routine, your body will respond.

It can be tempting to cruise through the same routine that you've always used. It worked up until this point, so what's wrong with it? By zoning out and letting yourself coast through the movements, you may be more likely to injure yourself. By failing to exert mental power along with muscular effort to perform exercises, you may be compensating or depending on synergistic muscles to help you complete the movements. This could eventually lead to altered movement patterns or even injury. When you change your routine, you're more focused on the movements—aka more likely to make smart choices and prevent yourself from careless mistakes that cause injury—and you're putting your mind to muscle. By focusing on the muscle you're intending to work, you're far more likely to feel (and see!) the results from your efforts. I've heard that Arnold Schwarzenegger used to visualize enormous mountains while he trained his biceps; I think it worked out well for him.

Master your motivation! Why are you working out? Why are you choosing to fuel your body with healthy foods? Keep this in mind along your journey, whether you're just getting started or continuing your current path. Do you need to bribe yourself a little along the way? (It's OK if you do! Treat yourself for consistency: "If I work out five days per week for this month, I'm buying a cute new workout top or a massage at the end of the month.")

My favorite motivation technique is creating an inspiration board at the beginning of each year. I make sure to include photos of my personal, health, and career goals, in addition to quotes and mantras to help me push through the challenging aspects. Pinterest is a fabulous spot to create an inspiration board, or you can do it the old-fashioned way with a stack of magazines, a pair of scissors, and a glue stick.

How do you change your routine?

Mode

What are you doing for your cardio? What tools are you using for strength training? Change it up. It could be something small, like transitioning from a treadmill to running outdoors, or something entirely different, like learning how to use kettlebells instead of dumbbells. Every few weeks, take a look at your schedule and see what mode changes can occur. Do you usually use dumbbells for your bent-over rows? Try a barbell instead. Changes, even small ones, keep the body guessing and facilitate fitness gains as well as fat loss.

Frequency

How often are you training? What time of day are your workouts? See if you can change up your frequency (making sure to allow at least one to two full days of rest or active recovery) or the time of day.

You may find that you're more energized after an early-morning workout, or that an afternoon strength session helps to curb the before-dinner sugar cravings.

Intensity

Are you working too hard, too often? Remember, less is more! Be sure to alternate workout intensities to allow for muscle repair, recovery, and general well-being. If you work to the max every day, your mind will feel as burned out as your body. Take a look at your workout intensities and determine when you can bump it up or dial it down a notch. As a general rule, avoid working out at the same intensity as yesterday.

Duration

Change up the duration of your workouts. When you usually do a 30-minute strength-only blitz, add in some cardio or HIIT intervals. Be sure to have some shorter days and longer days on your weekly schedule. (Nothing over an hour unless you're training for a fitness event. Seriously.)

Rest protocols

Change the rest time between sets as an easy way to keep your body guessing. Alternate between straight sets (with 30 to 60 seconds rest between each set) and circuit training (moving quickly from one exercise to the next with little to no rest between).

Getting more bang for your cardio buck

When I first had my daughter Livi, I didn't have the same amount of time to work out. I also didn't have the time or desire to work out as hard or as long as I once did. I wanted to be snuggling that baby! Of course, getting to the gym has helped me become more energized for my mom-ly duties and also provides an awesome blast of Zen time throughout the day. I have a good feeling you're busy, too, so here are some more ideas to get more out of your cardio session.

You should change up your cardio routine on a frequent basis—at a minimum, every four to six weeks.

Intervals and tempo work

For speed intervals, you can increase your speed to a challenging level for a set amount of time. Change up the intervals as often as possible. Play with speeds and length of time for each set. Some ideas:

- *Equal time ratios.* One minute hard, One minute easy. (Try the same with two or three minutes, or reduce the time to 45 or 30 seconds of each work-to-rest ratio)

- *Equal distance ratios.* One mile hard (FAST), One mile easy, repeat. You can choose any distance you like. A quarter-mile is a great starting point, and work your way up from there.

- *Single doubles.* One part speed or distance to two parts rest (or vice versa). You can do this with virtually any work-to-rest ratio, but endeavor to make it a little different each time.

- *Tempo Oreos.* The good stuff is in the middle. Start easy, and increase your speed in the middle of your workout. Hold it there for as long as you can manage and take it back down. An example: 10 minutes warm up, 20 minutes tempo push, 10 minutes easy/cool down.

- *Pyramids.* Accelerate the rate of speed for each speed drill. An example: Warm up for five minutes; increase your speed by 1.0 mile per hour, slow it down to your original pace; increase it by 2.0 miles per hour, slow down to original pace; increase by 3.0 miles per hour, return to original pace; increase by 3.5 miles per hour, return to original pace; 3.0 up, original, 2.0 up, original, cool down.

- *Hills.* By varying the incline of your walking or running workout, you not only add additional stressors, but also utilize different leg and core muscles. When you add the incline, it's important to remember that you're simulating an outdoor workout. When we're outside walking or running, we wouldn't be holding onto cacti or shrubbery, so you probably should avoid holding onto the handrails. Not only will you burn 30% fewer calories, but you'll be training yourself to walk or run inefficiently. To assist your climb up the hill, focus on engaging your core muscles and very slightly hinge forward from your hips. Endeavor to maintain a neutral spine position and avoid letting your shoulders creep up as the incline increases.

Some of my favorite ways to incorporate hills:

- *Hill challenge.* For this one, I'll increase the incline every 30 seconds to one minute until I can't take it anymore. When I get to the highest point, I hold it for at least two minutes and then gradually decrease the resistance. This is a killer glute workout!

- *Pyramid hills.* Find a starting incline and alternate between that original incline and a higher incline for each round. Decrease using the same method. For example, warm up at a moderate pace and incline, then add 2.0% incline and hold it for a minute (maintaining the same speed). Go back down to your original incline, hold for a minute, and then increase by 4%, hold, then back to your original incline. Continue this pattern for as long as you can maintain it, then, following the same method, make your way back down the hill.

Musical cardio

This is my all-time favorite cardio trick, but the #1 necessity is a killer playlist. Find a playlist that pumps you up, and be sure to include a mix of slower and faster songs. During the slow songs, visualize them as hills and chances to use hill challenges. Increase the resistance according to the music, or play fun games, like for every time the artist repeats a word, add resistance. (You'll hate that word by the time the song is over!) Use up-tempo songs for speed. During each fast-paced chorus, crank up your speed and use it as a sprint. Recover during the verses.

Use your entire body

The most effective cardio methods are ones with functional purposes (you walk and run in everyday life, but would you ever make an elliptical-shape motion with your feet? … just sayin'), and exercises that utilize your entire body: upper, lower, and core. If you want to get an efficient and quick workout, you need to challenge yourself. I think the best options are running/walking, jumping rope, rowing, plyometrics, and functional cardio, including calisthenics.

Put the magazine, eReader, tablet, smartphone, *everything* away

I'm sorry to say it, and I love reading on cardio equipment just as much as anyone, but *if you're short on time and want a quick workout, you need to focus and put the reading away.* While it's an enjoyable way to pass the time, when you can read or focus on something else entirely, you're not giving 100% to your workout. Of course, reading on the treadmill is a thousand times better than not going to the gym at all, but if you're looking for results and don't have a ton of time (to waste), you need to challenge yourself. Remember: no challenge, no change. If you're looking for a distraction during your workout, use a crazy awesome playlist instead. Audiobooks are also fun for longer, steady-state cardio, but I don't find them to be as motivating for killer short-duration workouts. Find out what pushes your workout buttons, and put the distractions away.

How to change your strength training routine

Add more weight

It seems like an obvious point, but how often are you really pushing the weight? If you've been lifting 8-pound dumbbells for your biceps curls for five years, I have a shocker for you: you can probably increase the weights. (And lifting weights will not make you bulky, I promise. Women do not have the hormonal makeup for that to occur, and every time a woman thinks that weight training will make her bulky, a fairy falls down dead.) A good way to gauge your challenge weight for exercises is how you feel at the end of each set. If you're not feeling challenged toward the end of each set, you could be working harder. Remember, it's all about efficiency! You can spend a lot of time lifting easy weights, or less time lifting challenging weights. I'd definitely suggest rolling with the latter.

Experiment with unstable surfaces and balance challenges

An easy way to add strength progression and target your internal core stabilizers is to change the surface of your workout. An excellent option is to use a physioball—perfect for chest presses, single-leg squats, and back extensions—or to perform the strength movement standing on one leg. A single leg deadlift is far more challenging than a regular ol' lift, and you'll also get a bonus core workout.

Add cardio blitzes to your routine

Every few sets, add in a heart-pounding cardio move, such as burpees, high knees, a short run (or run in place with high knees), vertical jumps, jumping rope, or squat jumps. Not only will this strategy add more excitement to your workout, but it will also increase your heart rate during your strength sets. This means that you can expect a higher overall calorie burn from your workout. It doesn't have to necessarily be high impact to increase your heart rate. If you're looking to minimize joint impact, try to increase the range of motion and dynamics in your exercises. By constantly shifting your center of gravity, the heart has to work harder. Beginners can try marching with high knees, or reaching up to the ceiling and down to touch the floor (with legs in a wide squat) as quickly as possible.

Change exercise selection

Make sure that you're not using the same moves each time you train a particular muscle group. For example, if you always do a standard biceps curl for your biceps, try a cable biceps curl, concentration curl, or hammer curl instead. If you're following the workouts in this book, you can substitute any exercise with another of the same type (like a reverse lunge with a kick instead of a suggested curtsy lunge). You'll be working essentially the same muscle groups in a different way.

Unilateral and bilateral movements

If it feels too easy doing both arms or both legs at the same time (for example, a biceps curl), try one at a time. Really increase the weight and mentally focus on the muscles you're targeting. Mind to muscle! In many studies, research has determined increased results if you visualize your muscles tightening and strengthening throughout your workout. There's much to be said about focusing during that short time instead of zoning out to your iPod.

Try new set and rep techniques

Here are some of my all-time favorites:

- *Pyramids.* For this type of training, you should increase or decrease your weight or repetition amounts to your most challenging point, and bring it back down. An example for strength training would be to perform 8 reps of a movement, then 10, then 12, then 10, and then 8. My favorite way to use pyramid training is during cardio workouts. On the treadmill, I'll increase the resistance every 30 seconds to one minute, and when I reach the top of my mountain for the day (usually between 15% and 20%), I'll start to decrease the incline each minute until I get back down to my home base. Depending on how much time I have, I'll repeat that technique for the duration of my workout.

- *Drop sets.* For drop sets, you start off your set with a more challenging weight than you're used to, and substitute your regular weight when it becomes too heavy. A tricky thing? Your usual weight will feel SO much heavier, since your muscles are already fatigued. For example, I usually biceps curl 12 to 15 pounds. For a drop set, I'll grab 20 pound dumbbells and start to do my usual set of 12. I'll only make it through four or five biceps curls, and then grab my trusty 15 pounder and finish the remaining seven repetitions. My biceps are *en fuego* by the time the first set is over.

- *Circuits.* During circuit training, you move from one exercise to the next with little to no rest in between. You'll do one full set (10 to 12 reps) of one exercise and continue in the circuit, repeating the entire thing two to three total times. In circuit training, you torch calories and feel your metabolism elevated for the rest of the day. Metabolic circuit training increases your metabolism because it elevates your EPOC and is a time-efficient way to improve cardiovascular fitness, building strength and endurance. You will blast calories during circuit training because the cardio blasts elevate your heart rate during the strength portions. You're moving quickly the entire time!

- *Number games.* If you really want to get cheeky with your strength training, have a little fun with numbers. You can think of your own patterns and sets, but here are some favorites:

  - *2, 4, 6, 8, 10:* You'll choose a few exercises (such as push-ups, squats, squat jumps, walking planks, and burpees), completing them two times, then four, then six, and so on, all the way up to 10 reps for each one.

  - *10, 9, 8, 7, 6, 5, 4, 3, 2, 10 (did you catch that last one?):* Try this one with biceps curls, first starting with 10 reps, then 9, 8, and so on, until you finish with 10. It's a doozy!

- *Time yourself.* Go for 30 seconds to one minute of an exercise, completing as many repetitions as you can within that time set. For example, set your timer for one minute and crank out as many push-ups as you can complete with good form within that time period. Resting is OK! Take a short breather, and come back when you're ready.

- *Add static holds or small pulses between each set.* When you usually do 12 reps, try holding the hardest part of the movement for 12 seconds after your reps, or pulse the weight for 12 small movements to fully fatigue the muscle. Biceps curls is a "favorite" routine: 10 full biceps curls, then hold the left curl in a static position while completing 10 more reps with the right, then switch (so you're holding the right curl and performing the full movement on the left), and then do 10 pulses with both arms at the most challenging part of the movement (where elbows are bent at a 90-degree angle).

Have fun with it!

If you're changing something, your body is changing along with it. Number games are also an excellent way to keep boredom at bay. (Poet, and I know it.)

How to avoid the dreaded plateau

You know the story: You're working hard with a new routine, killing it at the gym, eating clean, and seeing amazing results from your hard work. Then, out of nowhere, *BAM!* The results stop. Isn't that a mean trick when that happens? Plateaus are usually the result of these two culprits:

1) *noncompliance to your prescribed plan, or*

2) *adaptation to your current routine.*

Here's what to do if you ever find yourself face-to-face with the dreaded plateau:

Evaluate your routine

When was the last time you changed something? Always keep your body guessing to avoid adaptation and keep things exciting. Follow any of the strategies in this chapter to spice up your routine. Also make sure that you're getting adequate rest. As I said before, exhaustion will hinder your results.

Are you overestimating calorie expenditure and underestimating caloric intake? This can happen when you've experienced a change in lifestyle or occupations, causing more sedentary time or too many restaurant meals. In order to continue losing weight/fat (if that's your goal), you need to be at a deficit, meaning that you're consuming less than you're burning. You may have to up your activity, slightly decrease your caloric intake, or a small combination of the two to kickstart the process. If you need help assessing your meals and nutrient intake, check with a local registered dietitian for advice.

Reassess your caloric needs

A lower weight indicates that you need fewer calories. At the same time, higher muscle density BURNS more calories. Get your basal metabolic rate (BMR) checked by a registered dietitian, personal trainer, or exercise physiologist, or calculate an estimation of your intake requirements.

Here's a simple method to get an idea of how much to consume:

Take your weight, multiply it by 10, and add your weight to this number. (For example, if you weigh 150, 150 × 10 = 1500 + 150 = 1650.) There are quite a few methods of estimating BMR, but I've found that this is the simplest method, and the easiest to remember. If you have access to BOD POD measurement, VO2 max testing, or hydrostatic weighing, by all means, go for it (!!!) as those methods will be more accurate, but this is an easy way to gauge your estimated baseline expenditure.

As I said before, I'm not a huge advocate of counting calories, but if you need to do it for a little while to bust a plateau, it's a potentially helpful technique. Avoid making it a long-term thing if you can; your sanity will thank you when you're able to go by intuition and true hunger cues rather than an arbitrary number. Also, as I mentioned previously, your calorie needs change each day, so aim to hit around the same average each week (with maybe some higher or lower days in the mix).

Write down your meals

I have a (lame) rhyme for you: if you haven't been tracking, you could be slacking. Of course you should enjoy treats and fun things every now and again—decadent foods help make the world go round— but it's easy to get into mindless habits that potentially hinder fitness and fat loss results. Start writing down what you're eating, even if it's just for a seven-day period, to get an idea of easy nutrition fixes. For example, you may be reaching for a sweet snack for an energy boost midafternoon, even though you may not necessarily be hungry.

Instead, you could do something else like take a short walk, a catnap, or enjoy a stretch or a cup of green tea. According to a 2008 study by the *American Journal of Preventive Medicine*, by journaling their food, study participants lost 18 pounds versus 9 pounds in a 12-week period.

Portion food out

Over time, it's easy for portion sizes to grow, especially when we're used to dining out often. Eat your food on a smaller plate (an 8-inch, salad-sized plate works well) and go for vegetables first. Also, try to avoid drinking calories (through sugary drinks and juices) to see if it helps to bust the plateau.

Take a workout vacation

It seems counterintuitive, but by giving your body a chance to fully recover and rest, you will likely start to see new results when you resume your routine. By doing this, you're allowing yourself to become slightly deconditioned, which will result in a higher calorie burn from the same routine that you might have completed a week or two earlier. Also, if you've been running on "empty," by taking a full rest and week off, you'll return energized and ready to give more to your workouts and healthy lifestyle.

Reassess your goals

Make sure that your fitness and health goals are SMART (specific, measurable, attainable, realistic, and timely) and set up small checkpoint goals along the way to larger, more daunting ones. For example, if you want to run a half-marathon but have not run before, start off with a 5K and work your way up from there. It may seem as if this would be obvious, but I've had many clients in the past make goals that were unrealistic for their time frame, which only set them up for disappointment. If you feel small successes along the way, you'll be even more motivated to go after that big, scary goal.

Move a little more throughout the day

A pedometer is fantastic motivation to make sure you're getting enough steps. Aim for at least 10,000 steps per day, and enjoy parking farther from the mall entrance, walks with your pup, or extra bursts of activity during work. Fitness trackers are also a fun option. Though they're like glorified pedometers, these trackers can provide valuable insight into habits and patterns. Many also track sleep data, which could significantly affect fitness goals.

Surround yourself with support

Finding a new support network can help bust a plateau. Sign up for a running group, join a new yoga studio, enlist some fitness-loving friends to join you in your goal, or get involved with a virtual community. I have some lovely blog reader friends if you ever want to stop by (fitnessista.com). We'd love to have you!

HIITing it while you travel!

One of the most challenging aspects of traveling frequently can be fitting in workouts. Thankfully many hotels have fitness centers, and you can also pack a pair of resistance bands, sneakers, and some athletic clothes in your suitcase. Here's how I keep fitness routines intact while traveling:

- *Add in airport workouts.* No, I do not mean lunging down the terminal—even though I'll totally admit that I've done it—but instead of plopping in a chair with a coffee, spend layovers walking around the airport. It's an easy way to get in low-key cardio and shaking out your legs between flights. The way I think of it: I'm about to spend multiple hours sitting and/or sleeping, so I might as well get in some activity in an otherwise sedentary day.

- *Use frequent exploring as your workouts.* Sometimes I don't do many traditional workouts on vacation, but instead spend much of the day walking around. This way, I still enjoy indulgent and new food, but figure that it balances out with the extra walking throughout the day. If you're traveling for work, try to explore in between meetings or walk with friends to your conference destination instead of cabbing it.

- *Start the day early.* Usually, if I'm with family, I don't want to interrupt the day's plans by taking a fitness class or getting in a workout. Instead, I'll wake up a little earlier while everyone else is asleep and get in my sweat session then. This way, I'm done for the day before the fun begins.

■ *Work out at the hotel gym.* Check out the fitness center for traditional cardio and strength options. Many gyms have at least a set of dumbbells, a treadmill or elliptical, and a stability ball. Get creative with your options and for a fast and efficient combo, alternate strength sets with .25 to 1 mile runs or power walks on the treadmill.

■ *If your hotel or the place where you're staying doesn't have a standard gym, you can easily get in a bodyweight or resistance band workout in the comfort of your own room.* Many of the workouts found in this book can be adapted for a hotel room workout. Instead of dumbbells, you can use resistance bands (which are compact and lightweight; perfect travel companions) or get creative by using a backpack as your kettlebell. Worried about creating noise for the room below yours? Stick to low-impact options or try a yoga podcast.

Some of my favorite (quiet) hotel room moves include:

■ Bodyweight squats (holding a backpack for extra weight)

■ Push-ups (for a decline push-up option, put your feet on the hotel bed, hands on the floor)

■ Plank and plank walks

■ Weighted twists, holding a backpack

■ Resistance band exercises (biceps curls, triceps extensions, lateral raises, chest presses, reverse flys, gluteus medius side-to-side walks (step on the band for resistance, hold onto the handles and alternate taking big steps and small steps to each side; cross the bands for extra resistance), overhead presses, and so on. You can use resistance bands for many traditional dumbbell exercises, and even add them for crunches and abdominal work.

■ Warrior 3 to half-moons

■ Side leg lifts

- Plié squats into a calf raise (perform a classic plié squat and on the exhale, as you rise up you'll come up onto your toes. Lower down and squat again)

- Wall squats (standing with your back against a wall, lower down into a squat position creating a 90-degree angle with your legs. Extend your arms out in front of you and hold as long as possible)

Pick three to five of your favorite moves, set a timer for 10 to 15 minutes, and move quickly from one exercise to the next (12 to 15 reps of each exercise) in a circuit. It's a quick, sweaty, and quiet hotel room option.

- *Seek out local fitness studios.* One of my favorite aspects of traveling is the chance to take a couple of new classes or attend yoga at a different studio. Many fitness centers offer introductory rates, so your first class is free or fairly inexpensive. If time allows, it can be a lot of fun to try something new and maybe find a new method or instructor you adore. When we go to NYC or LA, I absolutely HAVE to take a Physique 57 class. I also have a running list of new studios or classes I'd like to try if I'm traveling and get the chance.

- *Vacation motivation.* When I travel, I either feel completely inspired to stick with my routine, or the total opposite. I feel drained, womp womp, and want to lounge by a pool drinking out of a coconut. (Even if we're in a spot where the only coconuts are found at the grocery store.) If anything, this could be a great opportunity to recharge. Take some time off and enjoy it. Give your body the chance to rebuild and recover, knowing that you'll be able to HIIT it harder when you return.

Whatever you decide to do: don't stress about it. Remember that it takes two weeks to decondition the body. Unless you're going on an extended trip or vacation with no activity whatsoever, it's unlikely that your trip will entirely derail your fitness progress. If you don't find time for activity or workouts while you're out of town, focus on clean eating as much as possible while you're there. Nutrition is what's going to have the highest impact on physical results. Also, you're on vacation (even if it's a work trip!). Don't spend it stressing on exercise or healthy eating. Please read the following statement in your best Elle Woods voice: Stress releases cortisol. Cortisol makes your body hold onto fat. Relax!

Getting back in the game

If you've been out of the fitness realm, for any number of reasons, it can be daunting and overwhelming to get back in the game. One of the most challenging times for me was when I had a newborn baby and was given the clearance to start working out again. Even though I was active throughout my pregnancy and the midwife said it was "OK" to resume normal activity, I didn't feel ready. I was so exhausted and dealing with anxiety and breastfeeding issues, I knew that the time would be better utilized for sleeping purposes. So that's what I did. I took some time to rest, enjoyed snuggling my new baby, and very slowly got back into the swing of things. I started with walking, which eventually turned into running, then strength training, and then HIIT workouts.

Here are some tips if you're getting started (again) after recovering from an injury, childbirth, or hiatus of any sort.

- *Don't expect to pick up where you left off.* The body becomes deconditioned after two weeks off from exercise. It's easy to think of this is a "bad" thing, but in reality, it can also be beneficial. Anything you do is considered new to the body, and you'll also experience a higher calorie burn from the same efforts you previously completed.

- *Make sure you have the "OK" from a doctor to resume normal fitness activity.* I hurt my knee by falling down the stairs in our house—I missed a step carrying a load of laundry and went sledding on my back all the way down—and ended up with an inflamed and angry knee. Running started to become painful, and when I told the doc that everything else felt fine, she said, "Well, don't run." I took 12 weeks off, which was miserable, and as soon as I got permission to start running again, I was able to gradually increase my mileage sans pain. Those doctors, they really know what they're talking about sometimes! Even though you may be tempted to resume activity early, it's not worth it. You could injure yourself further and end up out of the game for much longer than you'd originally anticipated.

- *Build up slowly.* Make your workouts purposefully too easy until you become comfortable with the motor and muscular processes again. Once you feel good with the standard movements, you can experiment with additional stressors like speed, incline, balance, and weight.

- *Be patient with yourself.* When I first got back into fitness after having a baby, I looked at pictures and thought I'd never be as strong or as lean as I once was. But I'm stronger now, leaner than I've ever been, and I feel proud of the fact that I'm able to make fitness a part of my life while also enjoying my role as a mama. Working out helps provide some sanity and "me time" throughout the day, and it also facilitates playing with my little girl. If I didn't take care of my health, I wouldn't be able to have dance parties, chase a soccer ball around the yard, or carry my 30-pound human kettlebell. Along your journey, stay mindful of the reasons why you want to take care of yourself. And now I'll also cliché-ly say that *fitness is a journey*. It will change and evolve as you continue to learn new techniques and adapt to various activities. Enjoy it!

"What comes easy won't last. What lasts won't come easy." You need to work and be consistent for results that will stick. The time will pass anyway! Would you rather look back a few months from now and be amazed by your accomplishments, or find yourself exactly where you are now? You can do it. At the same time, *be patient with yourself*. A lifestyle change doesn't happen overnight; start with small, maintainable goals and build up from there.

Leave your judgment hat at home

I know that when you're getting started on a fitness journey or revamping your routine, it can be tempting to tell everyone about it. It's working for you, so why not share the word? Also, I know what it feels like to be worried about people you love when they make unhealthy choices. Here's the thing: *if they want to make a change, they have to want it for themselves and make the decision on their own. No matter what you say, they're going to have to find their own internal motivation to make it happen.*

There have been too many times I've started to train clients and realized that they wanted a trainer to say they had a trainer, but they weren't ready to make significant changes. The best I could do was to lead by example, make their workouts enjoyable during the times we met, and try to be as encouraging as possible. If you find yourself in a similar situation, a winning strategy is to share the love and lead by example. Share some healthy treats you made, invite them on fitness-y dates (like checking out a new yoga class), but save the preaching and the judgment. If anything, they'll take notice of your energy, clear skin, and physical improvements, and may be inspired to make some healthy changes. *And if not, it's not on you.*

Chapter 5

More HIIT Workouts

Here are some more workouts and strength/cardio circuits, all of which can be completed in less than a half-hour. All of these workouts can be completed with a pair of dumbbells and your own body weight.

Cardio

HIIT

Bodyweight HIIT blitz

WARM-UP	
Moderate cardio	5 minutes
BODYWEIGHT HIIT BLITZ	
20 minutes	
40 seconds HARD	
20 seconds recovery	
For each exercise, do as many reps as possible within 1 minute	
Bodyweight Squats	
Jump Squats	
Jumping Jacks	

(continued)

BODYWEIGHT HIIT BLITZ (*continued*)
Air Jacks
High Knees
Burpees
Lateral Lunge to Basketball Throws (right side)
Lateral Lunge to Basketball Throws (left side)
Mountain Climber to Plank Walks
Jumping Planks
Jogging in Place
Jumping Rope (or High Knees)
Squats
Jumping Rope (or High Knees)
Jumping Squats
Jumping Rope (or High Knees)
Burpees
Jumping Rope (or High Knees)
Mountain Climbers
Jumping Rope (or Tuck Jumps)
COOL DOWN

HIIT scrambler

HIIT SCRAMBLER		
Time	Speed	Incline
0:00–5:00	Moderate speed	At least 2.0%
5:00–10:00	30 seconds HARD 30 seconds easy	Maintain incline
10:00–12:00	Keep speed at recovery zone	Increase incline by 5%
12:00–16:00	1 minute HARD 1 minute easy	Decrease incline to at least 2.0%
16:00–26:00	.25 mile HARD .25 mile easy	Maintain incline
26:00–28:00	Bring speed back to recovery zone	Climb the hill! Meet or beat what you did last time
28:00–30:00	Slow down and recover	0.0%–2.0% easy

Pyramid HIIT

PYRAMID HIIT		
Time	Speed	Incline
0:00–5:00	Easy	2.0%
5:00–10:00	30 seconds HARD 30 seconds easy	

(continued)

PYRAMID HIIT (continued)		
10:00–16:00	1 minute HARD 1 minute easy	Maintain incline
16:00–20:00	2 minutes HARD 2 minutes easy	Maintain incline
20:00–26:00	1 minute HARD 1 minute easy	Maintain incline
26:00–30:00	15 seconds HARD 15 seconds easy	Maintain incline
COOL DOWN		

Track work HIIT

Take it outside! Check out a local gym or school to use their track, or map out a 400-meter route in your neighborhood.

WARM-UP	
Moderate cardio	5 minutes
TRACK WORK HIIT	
15–25 minutes max 400 meters sprinting 400 meters easy	
COOL DOWN	

Steady state

Steps:

1) Choose your preferred cardio method. This could be a run, power walk, jog, bike ride, dance class, or cardio DVD (dance, kickboxing, step, etc.). If you're at the gym, or have cardio equipment at home, you could also use the Stairmill, treadmill, indoor rowing machine, or spin bike.

2) Warm up for five minutes at easy to moderate intensity

3) Determine how long you want to work out. Anywhere from 20 to 60 minutes is beneficial for a steady-state workout. Find a steady, moderate pace that you can maintain. If you're training with a heart rate monitor, endeavor to keep your heart rate in the range of 70% to 85% of your max heart rate.

4) Feel free to change up your speed or resistance during the workout, but be sure that you are not doing true intervals (breathless bursts of energy) on consecutive days. I like to gradually increase my speed, finishing at my fastest pace and then cooling down. This allows me to become accustomed to faster speeds and boost power during my workouts when I feel tired (an awesome strategy for racing). No matter what you decide to do: change it up on a regular basis. Try different modes, methods, and cardio durations to keep things exciting and keep your body guessing.

5) Cool down (five minutes) and then stretch if you'd like.

WARM-UP	
Moderate cardio	5 minutes
STEADY STATE	
20–60 minutes	
Heart rate at 70%–85%	
COOL DOWN	

Hills

You can perform hills in almost any mode of cardio. Increase the intensity and play around with it from there.

Rolling hills workout

ROLLING HILLS WORKOUT		
Time	Speed	Incline
0:00–5:00	Warm up, moderate speed	At least 2.5%
5:00–7:00	Moderate speed (RPE 6)	Increase your incline to a challenging level
7:00–10:00	Increase speed (RPE 7-8)	Decrease incline back to 2.5%
10:00–12:00	Decrease speed (RPE 6)	Increase incline; meet or beat last time
12:00–15:00	Increase speed (RPE 8)	Decrease incline to 4%
15:00–17:00	Decrease speed (RPE 7)	Increase incline by at least 2%
17:00–20:00	Increase speed (RPE 8)	Decrease incline by 2%
20:00–25:00	Increase or maintain speed	2.5% (incline homebase)
25:00–30:00	Moderate–easy (cool down)	0%–2.5%

Burn it out hill workout

BURN IT OUT HILL WORKOUT		
Time	Speed	Incline
0:00–5:00	Easy–moderate, warm-Up	2.5%
5:00–10:00	Increase speed to RPE 6	Increase incline at least 1% every 30 seconds
10:00–12:00	Maintain speed	Maintain highest Incline
12:00–15:00	Increase speed to RPE 8	2.5%
15:00–25:00	Decrease speed to RPE 6	Increase incline at least 1% every 30 seconds
25:00–28:00	Increase speed to RPE 8	Maintain highest incline
28:00–30:00	Decrease speed to easy, slow	0%–2.5%
COOL DOWN		

Cardio mountain

WARM-UP		
Moderate cardio	5 minutes	
CARDIO MOUNTAIN		
Time	Speed	Incline
5:00–15:00	Increase your speed every minute	Increase the incline every 30 seconds
15:00–20:00	Maintain highest speed	Maintain highest incline

(*continued*)

CARDIO MOUNTAIN (*continued*)		
20:00–25:00	Decrease your speed every minute	Decrease the incline every 30 seconds
25:00–28:00	Bring speed up to your maximum and maintain	Low incline
28:00–30:00	Slow down	Gradually decrease your incline

Booty blasting walking workout

BOOTY BLASTING WALKING WORKOUT		
Time	Speed	Incline
0:00–5:00	3.8–4.2 miles per hour	Start at 4.0% and increase to 7.0%
5:00–15:00	Maintain speed	Increase incline by 0.5%–1.0% every 30 seconds
15:00–18:00	Maintain speed	Maintain highest incline
18:00–20:00	Maintain	Decrease incline to 2.0%
20:00–28:00	Alternate between 30 seconds FAST walking and 30 seconds easy walking	Maintain at 2.0%
28:00–30:00	2 minutes FAST walking	Maintain at 2.0%
COOL DOWN		

2, 4, 6, 8, 10 Treadmill Workout

WARM-UP		
Moderate cardio	5 minutes	
2, 4, 6, 8, 10 TREADMILL WORKOUT		
Time	Speed	Incline
0:00–2:00	Steady pace	2.0%
2:00–6:00	Steady pace	4.0%
6:00–12:00	Steady pace	6.0%
12:00–20:00	Steady pace	8.0%
20.00–30:00	Steady pace	10%
COOL DOWN		

HIIT and steady

For this method, warm up, and then complete your HIIT rounds following any of the suggested ratios (1:1 or 1:2, distance or time based) for a set amount of time. After your HIIT, perform easy steady state (50% of your max heart rate) for the same amount of time. Here are some examples (increasing in difficulty):

Example 1

WARM-UP	
Moderate cardio	5 minutes
HIIT	
10 minutes	
1 minute HARD	
2 minutes easy	

(continued)

Example 1 (*continued*)

STEADY STATE
10 minutes
Heart rate at 50%
COOL DOWN

Example 2

WARM-UP	
Moderate cardio	5 minutes
HIIT	
10 minutes	
30 seconds HARD	
30 seconds easy	
STEADY STATE	
10 minutes	
Heart rate at 50%	
COOL DOWN	

Example 3

WARM-UP	
Moderate cardio	5 minutes
HIIT	
15 minutes	
30 seconds HARD	
30 seconds easy	
STEADY STATE	
15 minutes	
Heart rate at 50%	
COOL DOWN	

(I'm sure you get the idea! If you need more help setting up your HIIT ratios, be sure to refer back to pages 4 and 5.)

Strength

Upper body

Superset sweat: 25–30 minutes

WARM-UP	
Moderate cardio	5–10 minutes
SUPERSET 1	
3 rounds	

(continued)

SUPERSET 1 (*continued*)	
Biceps Curls	10–12 reps
Triceps Dips	15 reps
SUPERSET 2	
3 rounds	
Assisted Pull-ups	10 reps
Bent-over Rows	12 reps
Push-ups	12 reps
SUPERSET 3	
3 rounds	
Upright Rows	12 reps (heavy)
V-ups	12 reps
COOL DOWN	

Upper body jump and burn circuit: 30 minutes

WARM-UP	
Jumping Rope	5 minutes
Push-ups	10 reps

Bodyweight Squats	10 reps
Plank	1 minute
UPPER BODY JUMP AND BURN CIRCUIT	
Push-ups	1 minute
Upright Rows	12 reps
Biceps Curls	12 reps
Jump Rope HIIT	2 minutes 15 seconds HARD 15 seconds easy 4 rounds
Bent-over Rows	12 reps
Chest Presses	12 reps
Triceps Dips	1 minute
Jump Rope HIIT	2 minutes 15 seconds HARD 15 seconds easy 4 rounds
COOL DOWN	

Upper body blitz

WARM-UP	
Moderate cardio	5 minutes
UPPER BODY BLITZ	
15 minutes Complete as many rounds as possible	
Push-ups	15 reps
Triceps Dips	15 reps
Assisted Pull-ups OR Bent-over Rows	15 reps
Burpees	10 reps
COOL DOWN	

Arm burner
Note: Can be used after cardio (if you did not do arms yesterday!)

WARM-UP	
Moderate cardio	5 minutes
ARM BURNER	
15 minutes	
Upright Rows	15 reps

Hold arms in upright row position and drop one at a time, alternating	15 reps
Hold arms in upright row position and pulse	15 reps
Bent-over Row and Triceps Extensions	12 reps
Triceps Extension Pulses	12 reps
Hold Row Position	15 seconds
Biceps Curl Countdown	10, 9, 8, 7, 6, 5, 4, 3, 2, 10
AFTER ARM BURNER	
Biceps Curls	1 minute
Plank	1 minute
COOL DOWN	

Guns for days workout

WARM-UP	
Moderate cardio	5 minutes
GUNS FOR DAYS WORKOUT	
3 rounds	
Biceps Curls, Heavy	15 reps
Triceps Extensions	12 reps
Push-ups	15 reps

(*continued*)

GUNS FOR DAYS WORKOUT (*continued*)	
Bent-over Rows Challenge: do one leg rows or stand on a BOSU balance trainer	15 reps
Lateral Raises	15 reps
Plank	1 minute
COOL DOWN	

Lower body

Lean leg burner

WARM-UP	
Moderate cardio	5 minutes
LEAN LEG BURNER	
3 rounds	
Lunges (right)	12 reps
Lunges (left)	12 reps
Jumping Lunges	1 minute
Squats	12 reps
Squat Jumps	1 minute
COOL DOWN	

Booty blast circuit

WARM-UP	
Moderate cardio	5 minutes
BOOTY BLAST CIRCUIT	
3 rounds	
Curtsy Lunges (right side)	12 reps
Squats	12 reps
Hold Your Squat	12 breaths
Squats	12 reps
Curtsy Lunges (left side)	12 reps
Single Leg Deadlifts	12 reps on each side
Bridge	30 seconds
COOL DOWN	

Push combos

Push combo #1

WARM-UP	
Moderate cardio	5 minutes
CIRCUIT 1	
3 rounds	
Overhead Presses	12 reps
Triceps Kickbacks	12 reps
Chest Presses	12 reps

(*continued*)

Push combo #1 (*continued*)

REST	
30 seconds – 1 minute	
Run or walk .25 mile	
CIRCUIT 2	
3 rounds	
Plank with Lateral Raises	12 reps on each side
Push-ups	15 reps
Triceps Dips	15 reps
COOL DOWN	

Push combo #2

WARM-UP	
Moderate cardio	5 minutes
CIRCUIT 1	
3 rounds	
Overhead Presses	15 reps
Bent-over Triceps Extensions	15 reps
Push-ups	1 reps
REST	
30 seconds – 1 minute	
Burpees OR Wild Burpees	10 reps

CIRCUIT 2	
3 rounds	
Plank with Lateral Raises	10 reps on each side
Triceps Dips	15 reps
V-ups	1 minute
COOL DOWN	

Push combo #3

WARM-UP	
Moderate cardio	5 minutes
CIRCUIT 1	
3 rounds	
Upright Rows	15 reps
Overhead Triceps Extensions	15 reps
Bench Presses	15 reps
REST	
30 seconds–1 minute	
Your choice of bodyweight moves. (I suggest High Knees, Burpees, Squat Jumps with Rotation, and Jumping Lunges)	5 minutes 15 seconds HARD 15 seconds easy OR 40 seconds HARD 20 seconds easy

(continued)

Push combo #3 (*continued*)

CIRCUIT 2	
3 rounds	
Elevated Push-ups	15 reps
Triceps Dips	15 reps
Plank	1 minute
COOL DOWN	

Pull combos

Back and biceps burner

WARM-UP	
Moderate cardio	5 minutes
BACK AND BICEPS BURNER	
Assisted Pull-ups OR Bent-over Rows	15 reps
Biceps Curl Countdown	10, 9, 8, 7, 6, 5, 4, 3, 2, 10
Superman with Squeeze	1 minute
Single Leg Deadlift to Hammer Curls	12 reps on each side
COOL DOWN	

Pull muscle AMRAP

WARM-UP	
Moderate cardio	5 minutes
PULL MUSCLE AMRAP	
10 minutes Complete as many round as possible	
Assisted Pull-ups OR Bent-over Rows	15 reps
Biceps Curls, Heavy	10 reps
Single Leg Deadlifts	12 reps
Plank	1 minute
Renegade Rows (each side)	12 reps
COOL DOWN	

Legs and core

Total body circuit #1

WARM-UP	
Moderate cardio	5 minutes
TOTAL BODY CIRCUIT #1	
3 rounds	
Squats	12 reps
Hold Squats for Overhead Presses	10 reps
Renegade Row to Side Plank Lateral Raises	10 reps on each side
Burpees	10 reps
Side Lunge to Balance and Biceps Curls	10 reps on each side
Triceps Dips	15 reps
COOL DOWN	

Total body circuit #2

WARM-UP	
Moderate cardio	5 minutes
TOTAL BODY CIRCUIT #2	
3 rounds	
Lunge and Biceps Curl to Overhead Presses	12 reps, alternating legs
Single Leg Deadlift to Rows	10 reps on each side

Triceps Extensions	12 reps
Squats	15 reps
Push-ups	45 seconds
Plank (any variation)	45 seconds
COOL DOWN	

Endurance circuit

WARM-UP	
Moderate cardio	5 minutes
ENDURANCE CIRCUIT	
17 minutes For each of the following exercises, complete as many reps as possible in 1 minute before moving on to the next. When you complete your 5 minutes of work, rest for 1 minute, then do it again.	
Push-ups	
Squats	
Pull-ups	
Burpees	
Triceps Dips	
COOL DOWN	

Superset cardio circuit

WARM-UP	
Moderate cardio	5 minutes
SUPERSET 1	
3 rounds	
Biceps Curls	15 reps
Triceps Dips	15 reps
SUPERSET 2	
3 rounds	
Lateral Lunges (right)	10 reps
Lateral Lunges (left)	10 reps
Squats	10 reps
Calf Raises	10 reps
CARDIO BLAST	
5 minutes	
Start at an easy jog or walking pace with 5%–6% incline. Add 1% incline every minute until you have reached 5 minutes. (If you need to take it down before then, do it.)	
SUPERSET 3	
3 rounds	
Push-ups	12 reps Start in full plank and drop to your knees to finish if you need to.
Bent-over Flys	15 reps

(*continued*)

Superset cardio circuit (*continued*)

SUPERSET 4	
3 rounds	
Stability Ball Back Extensions	12–15 reps
Stability Ball Crunches	15 reps Hold a weight at the ends with both hands, keeping your arms close to your ears to make it more challenging.
CARDIO BLAST: SPRINTING	
5 minutes	
1 minute easy	
30 seconds HARD	
COOL DOWN	

Compound crusher

WARM-UP	
Moderate cardio	5 minutes
COMPOUND CRUSHER	
3 rounds	
Bent-over Single Leg Rows (right side)	12 reps
Plié Squat to Biceps Curls	12 reps
Jumping Lunges	1 minute
Overhead Presses	12 reps
Jumping Plank	30 seconds
Push-up to Side Plank	1 minute
COOL DOWN	

Functional mixer

WARM-UP	
Moderate cardio	5 minutes
CIRCUIT 1	
1 round	
Squats	1 minute
Push-ups	1 minute
Plank	1 minute Hold for as much of that time as you can. If you take a rest, come back when you're ready.
CIRCUIT 2	
3 rounds	
Running OR Bodyweight Cardio of Choice	400 meters OR 2 minutes
Biceps Curls (heavy)	10 reps
Dumbbell or Kettleball Swings	15 reps
Jumping Lunges	20 reps
CIRCUIT 3	
3 rounds	
Plié Squat to Upright Rows	12 reps

(continued)

CIRCUIT 3 (continued)	
Bent-over Rows	12 reps
Step-ups	10 reps on each side
Triceps Dips	15 reps on each side
COOL DOWN	

"Daaaaamn, girl!" Circuit

WARM-UP	
Moderate cardio	5 minutes
CIRCUIT	
3 rounds	
Squat Presses	12 reps
Burpees	15 reps
Lunge and Biceps Curls	10 reps on each side
Push-ups	15 reps on each side
Curtsy Lunge and Leg Lifts	10 reps on each side
V-ups	15 reps
Side Crunches	15 reps on each side
COOL DOWN	

Part Two

HIIT It! Diet

Chapter 6

HIIT It! Diet

We already know it's crucial to change up our workout routines on a regular basis, but it's just as important to alternate our eating. Our body gets used to the same fitness regimen, and guess what? It also gets used to eating the same amount of food, and the same types of food, at the same time, day in and day out. This is why many people who count calories judiciously initially lose weight and eventually plateau. Their body has adapted to its demands. Instead, you will learn the freedom of enjoying the fresh foods your body naturally craves and a numbers-free simple way to track food intake.

For our HIIT style of eating, all you need to remember is "HIIT": Healthy, Intuitive, Intermittent, and Track.

H = Healthy. This seems like an obvious requirement, but by "healthy," I'm insisting that you stick to whole foods if you want to see significant results from your efforts. Aim for food that has been untouched by the merits of science experiments, freaky food dyes, and preservatives. If you can, avoid food that came from a package, and if you find yourself looking for some packaged convenience options: read the ingredients. If you don't recognize something, put it down. If you don't recognize it, your body won't either.

Healthy eating habits to maintain: Providing adequate nourishment and fuels for our bodies; aiming for a mix of lean proteins, smart starches, and healthy fats; drinking plenty of water; eating the rainbow; and using our intuition when it comes to splurging, saving, and what our body may be telling us.

I = Intuition. When we "diet" or deprive ourselves of the foods we love, we tend to lose our intuitive eating abilities. No food is off limits. Sure, there are foods to emphasize for fitness gains and fat loss, but focus on the things you want to enjoy MORE often, instead of the foods that do nothing for us nutritionally but wrap our soul into the hug of an angel. To tap into your eating intuition, assess how badly you're craving or wanting the particular food.

Usually I can tell if I *really* want it—as in, I need to kill the whole plate full—or if I just want to taste it and have a few bites. Aim for a "grand scheme of things" approach, and try to eat clean most of the time so that when you eat "dirty," it's not a big deal. Look at your diet for the forest, not for the trees. Drinking adequate water (aim for at least 96 ounces per day) is a great starting point to avoid confusing thirst for hunger. Stop eating when you're full, and eat when you're hungry. It seems like a simple concept, but one that many of us have the ability to overcomplicate. If you look at a child, a child knows to eat when he or she is hungry, and stop when full, no matter how much food is left on the plate. If you feel guilty about leftovers—I despise wasting food!—freeze the rest or put it in the fridge for tomorrow's lunch.

While you're using your intuition, you may find that your food timing is more intermittent throughout the day. You may not eat breakfast until later because you realize you were eating out of habit, or that some days you intuitively consume more than others (which is a good thing). Follow your hunger cues and reach for whole foods first.

I = Intermittent. Try alternating your food intake and the timing of your meals, especially if you've been eating the same amount at the same time, day after day, for a long period. It's important to change things up with your eating, because you're able to get a variety of nutrients and keep things fun and exciting. Also, on certain days, you will need to consume more calories if you're more active, and less if you're more sedentary. By going with your intuitive cues instead of a schedule, you may find that your meal timing is more intermittent, and that's a good thing.

As far as higher consumption days go, in the fitness community, there's a little something called a "cheat day," but I don't love the negative connotation associated with that. *The only person you're cheating is yourself if you constantly nix foods you enjoy.* If I'm craving something particular, I eat it, and it's NBD. I enjoy the whole foods that energize me, and every now and again I have something glorious that makes me feel a little sluggish but tastes like heaven. By doing it this way, I've found that I don't really crave junk food; your body gets used to the energizing feeling, natural sweetness, and decadence found in nature's creations. Also, I've found that I enjoy the treat foods even more now that they're an occasional (but regular) thing.

One thing that helps to keep me from going overboard is physically jotting down my meals and snacks each day. This is a habit I had gotten out of when I had a baby—way too busy tracking diaper changes and feedings—but it is something that has worked and stuck with me for the long haul. My body has always thanked me, because writing things down helped me to make sure I was getting enough fresh produce, water, and nutrients to sustain my activity level while maintaining my energy levels and muscle gains. Now that my daughter is older, I've gotten back into jotting down meals and meal planning for the week. It's great inspiration to make healthy choices, fuel with produce, and ensure that critical nutrients aren't lacking. If I feel lethargic or sluggish, I can usually look back and see where I can make a small improvement.

T = Track. By tracking your food, you're able to more adequately assess how you're doing and what techniques work for you. It's also easy to determine little obstacles that may be standing in the way of your goals.

Each day, track your water intake (you need at least 96 ounces), fruits and veggie servings (aim for at least five), and how you feel (awesome, blah, motivated, tired, whatever). This will help you to assess any patterns that can be changed and small tweaks you can make to your current routine.

In my journal, next to my meals for the day, I write a few letters: C, F, P, N, T.

> *C = Carbs.* This includes starchy vegetables (white potatoes, sweet potatoes) and sweet vegetables (corn, carrots), legumes, fruits, beans, and grains (oats, brown rice, quinoa).
> *F = Fats.* All healthy fats including nuts (almonds, walnuts), seeds (hemp, chia, pumpkin seeds, sesame seeds), salmon, nut butters, and oils (ghee, coconut oil, grass-fed butter, flaxseed or walnut oil, olive oil).
> *P = Proteins.* Lean meat, seafood, and vegetarian protein sources (beans, etc.), including dairy. I personally don't eat a ton of dairy as it doesn't agree with me, but if it's something you enjoy as a part of your diet, keep it in. If you're not drinking fat-free dairy, it will double as a fat and protein.
> *N = Neutrals.* Green vegetables, salad greens, nonstarchy vegetables, and fruits (bell pepper, cucumber, artichoke, zucchini,

Daily Food Journal

	WHAT I ATE	**C**	**F**	**P**	**N**	**T**
BREAKFAST						
LUNCH						
DINNER						
SNACK/MINI MEAL						
SNACK/MINI MEAL						
TOTAL						

Water Intake

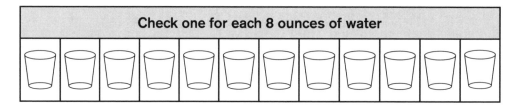

Check one for each 8 ounces of water

Fruits and Veggies

Check one apple for each serving of fruit or vegetables

How do I feel?

_____

_____

_____

_____

grapefruit, berries, green apple, onion, yellow squash, broccoli, and other cruciferous vegetables). No/low-calorie spices and seasonings are included here, too.

T = Treats. Anything not listed above, including sugary desserts and heavily processed and greasy foods.

As far as sugar goes, aim to sweeten your food with minimally processed lower-glycemic sweeteners including honey, dates, pure maple syrup, Sucanat, or coconut sugar. I also enjoy Stevia as a zero-calorie option, but many people dislike the slightly bitter taste. It's better to use a bit of real sugar than artificial sugars any day. Stay away from the blue and pink packets, mmm k?

C = Carbs
■ Beans and other legumes (pinto, kidney, black, cannellini, garbanzo)
■ Starchy vegetables (squashes, potatoes) and sweet vegetables (corn and carrots)
■ Amaranth
■ Barley
■ Brown rice
■ Corn tortillas
■ Oatmeal
■ Quinoa
■ Whole wheat products (check the labels to make sure that whole wheat is the #1 ingredient)
■ Fruits (bananas, kiwi, apples, melon, grapes, apricots, pears, peaches)

F = Fats
■ Fatty fish (salmon)
■ Tempeh
■ Full-fat dairy
■ Avocados
■ Nuts (peanuts, almonds, walnuts, cashews) and nut butters
■ Chia
■ Flax
■ Hemp
■ Oils (ghee, coconut oil, grass-fed butter, flaxseed or walnut oil, olive oil)

P = Protein
■ Chicken breast, chicken thighs
■ Eggs
■ Fatty fish (salmon)
■ Greek yogurt (goat or sheep milk yogurt are great options, too)
■ Lean turkey, dark turkey meat
■ Lean beef
■ Non-fat dairy
■ Protein powders
■ Seafood
■ Tempeh
■ Tofu
■ Avocados
■ Quinoa
■ Nuts (peanuts, almonds, walnuts, cashews) and nut butters
■ Chia
■ Flax
■ Hemp

N = Neutral
■ All green leafy vegetables
■ Artichokes
■ Asparagus
■ Bell peppers
■ Cucumbers
■ Cruciferous vegetables (broccoli and cauliflower)
■ Green beans
■ Lettuce
■ Onions
■ Zucchini
■ Citrus
■ Low sugar fruit (berries, green apples, grapefruit)
■ Condiments (mustard, vinegar, spices, garlic, ginger, herbs, zest)

As you can see, many foods double in certain categories. It can be a little tricky at first, but once you get the hang of it, it becomes second nature. Before you know it, you'll be able to look at a food and quickly eye the macronutrient components. This way, you'll be able to take a quick glance and assess how you're doing without getting out a calculator. It's much easier to skim through your notes for the day and realize you've had a lot of starchy and carb-heavy foods without enough protein or healthy fats in the mix.

There are also nutritional tracking apps—I'm a huge fan of MyFitnessPal—if that approach works better for your lifestyle. I'm an old-fashioned pen-and-paper girl, and writing by hand helps me track my macronutrients without too much calculation or emphasis on specific numbers. As I said before, it's more of a "grand scheme of things" approach.

If you do use an app, you may see that certain ratios work better for you and your goals. The general recommendation is 45% to 65% carbs, 20% to 35% fats, and 10% to 35% protein. For me, I feel and look my best around 50% carbs, 20% fat, and 30% protein. It's really a matter of finding the best combination for your body composition and lifestyle. Don't be afraid to experiment a little bit within the general guidelines, and determine what ratio helps you to feel your best while creating momentum toward your goals.

Eat like a PRO with protein and produce

There's a little saying I like to use on the blog: eat like a PRO. Emphasize *pro*tein and *pro*duce for the best fitness results, along with adequate water intake. First off, let's talk a little bit about protein, which tends to be overhyped in the fitness world. I think it's important to remember that while there are huge benefits in consuming protein, the average healthy person is easily able to get enough through a balanced diet without supplementation. I personally notice a difference when a meal contains a good source of protein; if it doesn't, I'm hungry about 14 seconds later. Not only will protein help to increase satiety, but it is also the building block to repair lean muscle tissue. Every cell in your body contains protein, and it's a critical component of skin, hair, muscles, and glands.

Grass-fed butter

I prefer grass-fed butter not only because of its taste, but because it's also a wonderful, healthy fat option. Grass-fed butter helps to raise our HDL ("good" cholesterol) and contains vitamin K-2, a rare nutrient that helps destroy calcification in our arteries. When purchasing any type of butter, check out the ingredients and make sure it's the real thing. Remember that a little goes a long way!

Coconut sugar

A low-glycemic sugar produced from the sap of cut flowers from the coconut palm. It has a rich flavor (not coconutty at all) and is especially delicious in baked goods. Find it online or at health food stores.

Sucanat

Sucanat (a clever merging of the words "sugar," "cane," and "natural") is whole, unrefined cane sugar. It's easier for the body to digest, as it's minimally processed, and boasts a warm, sweet flavor. It's an easy 1:1 switch for brown sugar. Many health food stores carry Sucanat and it can also be ordered online. Don't want to make the purchase? No worries; brown sugar works well in all of the recipes in this book (instead of coconut sugar or Sucanat).

Everyone has different protein requirements, depending on body composition goals/factors, sports performance goals, caloric consumption, and activity levels. A good rule of thumb is to make sure that each meal and snack has a little bit of protein. Some meals will yield higher protein content than others, but through a balanced diet of whole foods, it will equate to a sufficient amount throughout the day. Exercise increases the oxidation of amino acids (the building blocks of protein), so if you're active, you'll need more. Increasing the amount of protein in our diets can also help to prevent losing lean muscle while losing weight. The recommended protein intake is 10% to 35% of daily caloric intake, which leaves enough wiggle room for consideration with goals, personal factors, and satiety. According to the American Dietetic Association, here are some protein guidelines:

Activity Level	Grams of protein per kilogram body weight per day
Sedentary adult	0.8 (0.4 grams per pound)
Strength athletes	1.2-1.7 (0.5-0.8 grams per pound)
Endurance athletes	1.2-1.4 (0.5-0.6 grams per pound)

Now, onto the second part of the PRO mentality: produce! Fresh produce is important in a balanced diet because it has a low energy density (meaning little calories for the amount of food consumed) and high nutrient density (micronutrients like vitamins and minerals in addition to antioxidants). In research completed by Dr. Barbara Rolls, it was determined that people will eat the same weight of food, regardless of the total calories. This means that a one-pound salad (with a lower amount of calories) would equal the perceived satisfaction from a pound of pizza (much higher caloric toll).

When in doubt, choose whole foods

One of my friends has a great saying, "If it won't rot, don't eat it. It's not food." A good rule of thumb: if it came relatively unchanged from the earth, eat it; if it came highly processed from a factory, skip it. Because many of the nutrients from processed foods are stripped from the source and added back later, they tend to lack staying-power. Choose foods that will keep you satisfied for the long run, especially if you're busy and active, as many of you are!

Foods that have the ability to spoil are more easily broken down in the digestive process. This will leave more energy for other processes (like burning fat!) and help to prevent bloat. Not only are processed foods harder to digest, but they're also highly addictive.

Processed foods trigger the release of dopamine, which is the "pleasure" transmitter of the body. Find something else that gives you the same feel-good warm fuzzies, whether it's a walk outside, a chat with a friend, a manicure, or homemade juice. It can be a little challenging to strip your diet of processed food-like culprits, but once you do, chances are that you won't miss them. It takes 21 days to create a habit, so it can be advantageous to ditch these things cold turkey or eliminate them slowly over time, depending on your personal preferences.

Keep portion control in check

Aim to fill up your plate with mostly fresh produce, a little protein, and a little starch/grains.

Some easy portion guidelines:

- Meat/protein serving: The size of a deck of cards (4 ounces)
- Nuts and seeds serving: Cup your hand, and take whatever fits into your palm (¼ cup)
- Fruit serving: A fist (1 cup)
- Cheeses: Your pinky finger (1 ounce)
- Oils and dressings: Make a circle with your thumb and index finger and mentally "color" the circle with dressing (1 tablespoon)

Hydrate

It's very easy to mistake thirst for hunger, so if you're adequately hydrated, you won't get that "Am I hungry or thirsty?" mixed message. Drink water, even if you don't feel parched. Dehydration can lead to brittle hair and nails, sullen skin, and a cranky attitude. One of my friends taught me this trick: put 8 to 10 of your favorite little snacks, such as chocolate chips or berries, into a small dish. Enjoy one each time you have a large glass of water, so they act as hydration reminders plus being a bonus little treat. I also like to take a permanent marker to a large water bottle and mark when I should consume "x" amount of water. For example, by 10 a.m. I should have slammed at least 16 ounces. You could also be techie about it and set a silent phone alarm to remind you to drink every hour.

Also, if you're well-hydrated, it will be much easier to make smart food choices. When you're enjoying cocktails or wine with dinner, make sure to keep sipping water, too. Not only will this potentially stave off an embarrassing alcohol-induced moment waiting to happen, but it also helps to keep the dessert tray from making googly eyes at you.

Eat before you're starving

Whenever I wait until I'm too hungry, my good intention of a small snack or reasonable meal turns into stuffing myself as quickly as possible. By the time the amount of food I consumed catches up with me: zzzzzzz. I'm ready for a nap. You know that little hunger cue? (Mine is when my eyes start to look a little crazy—I kid.) Act on it before it turns into emergency mode.

Always have an emergency snack available

Have an emergency snack with you at all times. In my purse, I'll usually have some homemade trail mix, a bar, or at least an apple. This way if I find myself stuck somewhere and hungry, I have a smart choice I can depend on. It's much better than standing in line somewhere and having to hit up a vending machine or drive-thru. (For lots of healthy snack options, check out the upcoming chapter.)

Food combos to fuel your day

By having a general guideline to follow, it can make healthy choices much easier. Following is an example of food combinations and snacks I put together, which was approved by Registered Dietitian Anne Mauney, MPH, RD. It includes a nice mix of macronutrients, timing, and flexibility, which is ideal for a busy lifestyle. It's also based on my HIIT strategy of eating: snacks throughout the day, bursts of effort through planning and prepping, then reaping the rewards of your efforts throughout the week.

I set these combinations up similarly to how I fuel throughout the week, starting with five days of each week consisting of mini meals, which are like large snacks. They're enough to be totally satisfying without giving that sluggish, food-baby feeling. By snacking constantly throughout the day, it provides a steady stream of energy and delicious eats to fuel my activities.

Sample eating schedule

Breakfast: P, F, C (N optional)
Mid-morning snack: P, C (N optional)
Lunch: P, F, C (N optional)
Mid-afternoon snack: P (N optional)
Dinner: P, F, C (N optional)

So where's the "T"? It's not included up there, but can go wherever you feel like a treat. I try to keep the "Ts" around one to three servings per week if I'm working to achieve significant fat loss or fitness gains. When you're in maintenance mode, you already have an idea of how many treats you can enjoy in your routine while maintaining the goals you've accomplished. Sometimes a bit of something sweet is all I need, while on other occasions, it's the whole enchilada … or pizza cookie (see recipe on page 267).

When to splurge and save with food choices

In the proverbial bank of our body, in the end, weight loss is determined by food intake and outtake. Intake is the food we consume, and outtake is the fuel we use for everyday functions, activities, and exercise.

Sure, someone who eats 1800 calories of lean proteins, smart carbs, and healthy fats is going to look and feel entirely different than someone who consumes 1800 calories of refined sugars, white flours, and greasy foods. *However, in the grand scheme of things, weight is a matter of caloric intake and expenditure.* If you're trying to lose weight, you want to burn more than you're consuming. A safe rate of weight loss is 1 to 2 pounds per week. Since one pound of fat equates to approximately 3500 calories, a simple way to do this is to achieve a 500 calorie deficit each day during the week (500 x 7 = 3500), whether it's from exercise or food. This may sound totally obvious, but many people fail to realize how much they're burning (or not burning!) during the day. Your body needs enough fuel to sustain everyday activities, and if that doesn't happen it will kick into starvation mode and hold onto everything it can.

Remember, your body burns calories through the necessary processes *to live*. If you lay in bed all day, you'd burn a baseline amount of calories (also referred to as BMR, your basal metabolic rate). Not eating enough calories can be as hindering as eating too many. For this reason (along with at least 15 others), *I don't recommend counting calories*. It works well for many people, but I've found in my personal experience that it turns eating into too much of a math project. Eating should be enjoyable! I've found that by eating smaller meals with satisfying ratios (of protein, fats, and carbs) and allowing myself to enjoy treats, I was able to more easily lose the weight I gained after having our first baby. Instead of the yo-yo-dieting ways of the past, this simple method was the most effective; I was consistent with making whole and healthy choices for the most part, but still knew when I needed a treat night or to skip the gym to facilitate recovery.

Some of my strategies to decide whether to splurge or save with food choices:

Is it homemade? Usually if I want a dessert, this is a major decision factor for me. If someone made it with love, I want to try it. If a soulless factory machine made it, I don't seem to be as intrigued. Homemade stuff always tastes 100% better than the store-bought variety. For example: A plastic container of sugar cookies? Meh. Soft, homemade chocolate chip cookies? Yes, please.

Is it a special occasion or party? The same thing goes if it's a special occasion. I like to take inventory of what's available and go from there. If there's a large plate of crudités, beautiful salad, fruit, greasy pizza, and cake, I'll have salad, fruit, veggies, and cake, skipping the pizza. If the pizza looked amazing, I'd enjoy some and maybe have a little less cake (OK, and pick the frosting off my husband's. I'm a notorious frosting bandit). You have to assess what's "worth it for you" out of all of the choices, and if everything looks good, have a small bit of everything. I once read that Giada—you know the Giada I'm talking about—"tastes everything, but eats nothing." That's a fabulous party mentality to have. Enjoy little bits, and go back for more of what you really enjoy.

Am I hungry, thirsty, bored, stressed? I like to take a mental assessment of how I'm feeling if I start to go overboard (like with tortilla chips. I caaaan't stopppppp). Whether I'm eating junk food because I'm actually hungry, or if it's more of a "hot damn, this is salty and delicious!" Usually, just by taking a second to assess, it will at least encourage me to slow down a little. Food is fuel for the body. Of course, there are social aspects of food and it should be enjoyed, but I also try to stay mindful of the fact that it isn't a quick fix for feelings. If I'm stressed out, a brownie will only make me feel better for the 30 seconds I'm eating it. When it's gone, I'll likely still feel stressed.

Am I doing this out of habit? For a while, I got into the habit of having some chocolate each morning before my a.m. coffee. After a bit of time, I realized that I was still wanting chocolate throughout the day, and I wasn't even enjoying my morning chocolate habit. It was just that: a habit. I stopped doing it, and haven't missed it. Since then, I enjoy my afternoon chocolate or desserts much more than the handful of dark chocolate I sleepily ate while I waited for the coffee maker to wake up. I don't transition from zombie mode until my first cup of Joe is downed anyway.

What to order at a restaurant

When we're out and about, I have a few methods of navigating the restaurant menu.

Is it a special occasion or a new restaurant? Do I want to stick to my usual clean eats, or am I in the mood for something more decadent? If it's a special occasion, or I'm trying a totally new-to-me spot, I'll order something fairly indulgent and keep portion control in mind. Restaurant serving sizes are usually obscene, so I can plan on taking about half home for lunch the next day.

If I want to stick to clean eats (aka it's not a special occasion, date night, girls' night, or new/exciting restaurant), here's what I'll usually pick from the menu:

- *A salad.* I always like to have a salad with my meal, especially since it's a high-nutrient, low-energy-density food (whoa, that's a mouthful), and is a filling and healthy option. If you're checking out salad options on the menu, be wary of the ingredients and add-ins, as they can quickly make the salad as dense and fattening as a large greasy meal. Some things to watch out for: creamy, decadent dressings (ask for vinaigrette or the creamy dressing on the side), high-fat toppings (cheese, nuts, avocado: pick one you enjoy), sweets (such as candied nuts or dried fruits), or fried garnishes (nix these). Look for a salad option that's loaded with greens and fresh veggies, then add one high-fat delicious topping you love, a protein, and something sweet (such as fruit, berries, or dried fruit) if you'd like.

- *A protein-packed entrée.* Fish is usually a smart choice (go for baked, steamed, poached, or grilled), along with steamed veggies, brown rice, or sweet potato.

- *Pick two out of three: wine, bread, dessert.* For me, wine and dessert usually win. I like to share dessert, since I'm usually satisfied from dinner but want to try a couple of bites of whatever dessert the restaurant offers. If I don't see any desserts that sound particularly appealing, I stick with a glass of wine and call it a night.

I'll drink water with the meal and enjoy the company of those around me. Even though it's fun to check out a new restaurant spot, I'm usually there for the company more than the food. I soak in the experience and fun times with those I love; the meal is just the icing on the proverbial cake. It's easier to be mindful of portion sizes when you're having a lovely conversation and enjoying the whole experience.

I think it's worth mentioning that if you're at a restaurant and really want to try a certain menu option: GO FOR IT! If you order something you really don't want to eat ("I feel like I need to eat healthy so I'm going to order a salad, even though I really want pasta.") your meal will not be fulfilling and enjoyable to you. Also, you could end up overdoing it on cocktails, the bread basket, or dessert, since you didn't fully enjoy your entrée. Order what you want, but savor the bites and keep portion control in mind.

Some restaurant tips and tricks

- *Say it with a smile.* If you want to make a change to a menu offering, ask politely and tip well. Usually servers are used to making accommodations, especially if you ask with kindness. If you are unable to make a change to the menu, look for something

(continued)

grilled, roasted, or baked. Try to stay away from fried varieties and those decadent descriptive words like "creamy," "crispy," and "golden."

- *Remember the classic dinner combo, aka the "HIIT It dinner combo."* Most American restaurants will have a variation of protein, sweet potato (or extra veggies), and green veggies or a salad. Ask for grilled chicken or fish, steamed veggies, and sweet potato. This is my go-to restaurant order, which is especially wonderful with some lemon squeezed on top or some balsamic vinaigrette. Substitute greasy sides with steamed veggies, sweet potato, and/or a salad.

- *Mexican restaurants have a lot of healthy options!* Usually they'll have a version of a taco salad, which I'll ask for in a bowl instead of a shell, with no dairy (cheese or sour cream). Add guacamole and salsa for the dressing and it's a fantastic and satisfying meal.

- *Sushi restaurants.* Many sushi houses offer brown rice sushi or cucumber instead of rice. Pair it with edamame or a house salad, and try to watch your portions with the sushi rolls. Usually, I like to choose one plain roll (with fish and veggies) and one more decadent roll to share (with fried fish, avocado, crazy spicy stuff, whatever).

- *Sandwich shops.* Many sandwich stops have salad options or will make your sandwich on lettuce instead of bread. If you want a traditional sandwich, try a whole-grain option (the grainier, the better), a flatbread, pita, or wrap. In lieu of mayo, roll with mustard, hot sauce, and any veggies/condiments you enjoy. If you enjoy mayo or cheese on your sandwich, try asking for one or the other instead of both.

- *Asian restaurants.* Many places are happy to steam your entrée instead of frying. Ask for brown rice, protein, and veggies, and you're good to go. If you want to be cautious about the sauce, which can be obscenely high in sodium, ask for it on the side. Rolls wrapped in rice paper are also a great option in addition to soup and salad bowls. There are quite a few fried delicacies, too. If you want to go with something fried along with your clean meal (like a couple of fried wontons, which are deeeeelicious) just keep portion control in mind.

- *Pizza can be a fairly healthy option.* Ask for thin or whole-grain crust, lots of veggies, some chicken (if you like/eat poultry), and light on the cheese. Have two slices instead of the whole thing, and pair with a green salad.

- *Order dressings, heavy sauces, and calorie-dense toppings on the side.* You can also ask for "light dressing" so the chef doesn't get overzealous with his pouring skills. Lemon is also a great salad dressing option. Ask for a side of lemon, and squeeze some juice onto your meal for a fresh citrus kick.

- *Sharing is caring!* I love to order a large salad and an entrée or a couple of appetizers to share. I love sharing different meals at restaurants and this gives me a chance to try something new without the commitment of a full entrée.

Chapter 7

Snack Attack

I'm a huge fan of snacking throughout the day. It's a great way to keep energy levels stable, especially if you're gearing up for an important meeting or afternoon workout. It can be tricky to find healthy snacks on the go, so the best bet is to create fulfilling and portable options to have in your snack arsenal. Some people find that by snacking throughout the day, they have a steadier stream of energy. Others enjoy having larger meals within a shorter time period to give the body more time to digest. Find what method works best for you! I personally like to alternate based on how I'm feeling in addition to my activity level for the day.

No matter what strategy you decide to follow, planning and preparation make healthy choices much easier. Stock up on your snacks and staples for the week so you never find yourself in "emergency snack mode" (a scary moment for me!). A prepped Fitnessista always has a grab-and-go snack on hand, stashed in her purse or gym bag for late meetings, long commutes, or any time the snack attack hits. Keep reading for lots of great snack choices to have on-hand and can travel well.

Grocery staples

Here's a list of the foods I always have on hand that can easily create clean eating combinations to enjoy throughout the week.

Grains, nuts, and seeds
- Oatmeal
- Quinoa
- Brown rice
- Raw almonds

- Chia seeds
- Hemp seeds

Dairy
- Goat's milk Greek yogurt
- Goat's milk gouda or manchego cheese
- Grass-fed butter
- Organic eggs

Fresh produce
- Salad greens (I try to alternate these each week to get in a variety of nutrients and keep things exciting. Some faves include spinach, kale, Swiss chard, romaine, and broccoli slaw.)
- Berries (raspberries, blueberries, blackberries)
- Bananas
- A couple of seasonal items: apples, pears, kiwi, peaches, whatever looks fresh
- Sweet potatoes
- Zucchini and/or yellow squash
- Avocados
- Limes and lemons
- Garlic, onions, ginger, and fresh herbs

Pantry items
- Canned tomatoes
- Dried or canned beans
- Almond butter or sunflower seed butter (store in the fridge once opened)
- Local honey
- Pure maple syrup (store in the fridge once opened)
- Coconut oil

Condiments
- A variety of spices (staples: oregano, thyme, paprika, garlic powder, salt, pepper, cinnamon, alcohol-free vanilla extract)
- Hot sauce

- Dijon mustard
- Apple cider vinegar
- Balsamic vinegar
- Red wine vinegar
- Extra virgin olive oil
- Tamari or Nama Shoyu (or low-sodium soy sauce; store in the fridge once opened)

Tips for creating the perfect snack

Make your meals/snacks suit your workouts and lifestyle

Remember that you're not running a marathon in your sleep. Plan out your snacks so that you're getting enough protein to make it through the night and enough carbs to sustain energy for the day.

I remember the time I went to teach and take dance classes for the evening and realized, midway through my nightly four hours at the studio, that I hadn't had a single healthy carb that day. My jumps were sloppy and lackluster. A colleague asked if I had "a cold or something." The only carbs I'd consumed were from the sugar volcano in my morning latte, and in addition to a breakfast of eggs, a lunch protein bar, and deli salad, it wasn't enough. From then on, I made sure to get in a satisfying amount of fuel and brought snacks with me to enjoy between dance classes. My jumps improved dramatically. Focus on carbs before your workout, and protein and carbs afterward.

Emphasize protein with a little healthy fat or carbs to accompany it

A sugar buzz can be tempting, but it is a fake energy boost that often leaves me feeling zonked (and craving more of the sweet stuff) after reaching for a sugary snack. It's totally OK to enjoy a little dessert or treat every now and again, but for the most part, a satisfying snack should contain protein. I don't think meals should involve a calculator, which is why I avoid suggesting certain gram amounts, but for a satisfying snack, aim for mostly protein (P), with minimal fats (F) and few carbs (C).

Some of my favorite high-protein options

- **Steamed or boiled eggs.** I used to have the worst time boiling eggs. They'd be over- or undercooked every time! So my chef brother taught me the steamer basket trick, and now I steam eggs in a steamer basket instead of boiling them. Just 15 minutes to perfect eggs! If you are an egg boiling wizard, you can totally boil them instead.

- **Protein "fluff."** One tablespoon of almond butter (or any nut butter), half a scoop of protein powder, a little cinnamon, and enough almond milk to thin it out (about 2 tablespoons). Heat in the microwave for 20 seconds, stir, and serve on top of fruit, toast, or a whole-grain waffle.

- **Amazeballs.** (see recipe on page 190)

- **Snackable smoothie.** (see recipe on page 191)

- **Deli wrap.** Tofu, turkey, or tempeh rolled up with veggies, a slice of your favorite cheese, Dijon mustard, hot sauce, and lettuce. One of my favorites is asparagus wrapped with turkey and goat cheese, baked in the oven or toaster oven.

- **Fruit and cheese.** Goat cheese is lovely crumbled onto sliced pear, or try some sliced cheddar on an apple.

- **Homemade trail mix.** In a large bowl, combine 1 cup of your favorite nut/seed combo, a quarter cup dried fruit, and a quarter cup dark chocolate chips. Divide into four servings and store in baggies for an on-the-run snack.

- **Protein bars.** There are a lot of health food bars on the market, so here are some things I like to keep in mind while choosing mine. First, check the ingredients. Is there anything you don't understand? Skip it. Be wary of soy protein isolate, added/fake sugars, and high-fructose corn syrup. Many of my favorite bars contain fruit, nut butter, nuts, and maybe some vegan or egg white protein. Simple is better. I like Vega Sport, GoodOnYa, KIND bars, RX bars, and Pure Bars as they contain simple whole ingredients and taste delicious.

- For a quick and easy homemade bar, grind up 1 cup almonds, 10 Medjool dates, a quarter cup of chocolate chips, a quarter teaspoon cinnamon, and a pinch of sea salt in a food processor. After a soft dough forms, press flat in a large airtight container and store in the fridge before cutting into four to six bars.

- **Fruit or vegetables with nut/seed butter.** Take your favorite fruit or veg and serve with 1 heaping tablespoon of nut/seed butter. I love strawberries dipped in cashew butter. Try apple dipped into sunflower seed butter for a delicious treat. Carrots are surprisingly yummy dipped in almond butter. If you're going to be on the go, pick up some single-serve packets of nut butter. They're easy to toss in your purse with a piece of fruit!

- **Pizza toast.** One slice of toast with cheese of choice and marinara sauce.

- **Egg puff.** Spray a bowl with nonstick spray, add an egg, whisk with a fork, and microwave for one to two minutes. (If you hear the egg make a "pop!" sound, check it, and continue to cook as needed.)

- **Easy protein pancake.** One egg, one scoop of protein powder, and one-half of a banana, whisk, and cook like a pancake.

Some of my favorite veggie-friendly protein options

A commonly spouted nutrition myth is that vegetarians don't get enough protein. While animal protein sources may be the first to come to mind, it's extremely easy to get enough macronutrients and thrive on a plant-based diet. To get adequate protein, ensure that you're consuming sufficient produce, nuts, seeds, healthy fats, and eggs (if they're a part of your diet). I do think that we're overcarbed as a society—refined carbs are served with virtually everything—and I am guilty of participating in the "peanut butter and bread diet" in one of my many forays into vegetarianism. I think the key to being a smart, energized veggie is to research nutrition, get plenty of fresh produce (VEGetarian! Not CARBitarian), and talk to your doc about necessary supplementation.

- **Beans/legumes:** Not only are beans inexpensive and filling, but they're also extremely versatile. Beans make lovely salad toppings, dip components, wrap fillings, and stir fries. Edamame has 17 grams of protein per quarter cup serving; lentils have 18 grams of protein per cup; pinto beans, black beans, and garbanzo beans all have around 15 grams of protein per cup (for around 250 calories).

- **Nuts and seeds:** Nuts and seeds provide a delicious dose of healthy fat in addition to protein. They can be made into vegetarian nut pâtés, faux meat scrambles, or patties, ground into meal or made into nut/seed butter. Per 10 gram serving, pumpkin seeds contain 2.7 grams of protein, sesame seeds yield 2 grams, almonds contain 2 grams, and pistachios contain 2.4 grams.

- **Green veggies and leafy greens:** Green veggies and leafy greens are a surprising source of protein. They're the quintessential base for salads and are also delicious juiced, roasted, stir fried, baked into chips, or blended in a smoothie. (For smoothies, I recommend kale and spinach … not so much the zucchini or asparagus.) Asparagus, broccoli, and artichokes each contain 3 grams of protein per serving.

- **Sea vegetables:** These contain about 3 grams of protein per serving and include iron, iodine, and vitamins C and B2. They have anti-inflammatory properties and are high in cancer-fighting phytonutrients. Sea vegetables such as kelp, kombu, dulse, nori, arame, and wakame yield a salty flavor and are found in the international aisle of most grocery stores. Try using nori as a sushi wrapper, or sprinkling some dulse or arame on your salad bowl or stir fry. They also make lovely marinated salads and soups. Simply rehydrate in water, drain, and season to your preference.

- **Nutritional yeast:** Nutritional yeast is one of my favorite vegetarian cheese substitutes. It's especially delicious sprinkled onto salads, pizza, popcorn, and eggs. It has a nutty, cheesy taste to it, and is extremely high in protein. One 80 calorie serving provides 8 grams of protein!

- **Faux meat products:** I don't usually recommend these, as they're highly processed and soy-dominant (soy is one of the most common GM (genetically modified) crops) but if you like them and they work for you, continue to enjoy in moderation. The ones I tend to enjoy the most are the ones including whole foods, like Sunshine burgers and sprouted tempeh creations.

- **Vegan-friendly protein powders:** There are some fantastic vegan protein powders on the market, including Vega, a plant-based blend, and Sun Warrior, which is made using brown rice. Most vegetarian or vegan protein powders will contain 15 to 22 grams of protein per serving.

Nutritional yeast

This deactivated yeast is a powdered supplement and boasts a "cheesy" flavor. It's an ideal dairy substitute for vegetarians and vegans, especially since it's high in B vitamins and protein. Most health food stores carry nutritional yeast in larger bins or in the bulk section. I recommend getting a small amount from the bulk bins until you become accustomed to the taste and want to invest in a larger bin. I especially enjoy nutritional yeast on eggs, pasta, and salad and to make cheese-like sauces, like the one that coats my beloved kale chips.

Protein powder

This is a matter of personal preference, as there are a vast amount of protein varieties. You can try whey protein, which is dairy-based, or experiment with vegetarian (egg white) or vegan (brown rice, hemp, pea, soy, etc.) protein. I personally enjoy egg white protein for yogurts and smoothies, and brown rice protein for everything else. You can find protein powder at health food stores and specialty nutrition stores. A little tip: many stores offer sample sizes of protein that you can try before committing to the full-sized tub.

Standby snacks

- Amazeballs
- Snackable smoothie
- Perfect protein pancakes
- Turkey lentil muffins
- Egg and veggie muffins
- Chicken spring or nori rolls
- Cinnamon quinoa muffin tops
- Banana almond muffins
- Chocolate protein bars
- Pumpkin chocolate chip muffins

Amazeballs (*P, F*)

Makes 5 large or 10 small protein balls

> ¼ cup dry ingredients (such as protein powder, oats, almond meal, or unsweetened coconut. I usually use 2 Tb each of protein powder and coconut.)
>
> ¼ cup mix-ins (use any combination of chocolate chips, dried fruit, nuts or seeds, citrus zest, and juice)
>
> 2 Tb nut butter of choice (such as almond or cashew butter)
>
> 2 Tb pure maple syrup
>
> ¼ tsp vanilla extract
>
> Pinch of sea salt
>
> Pinch of cinnamon (optional)

1. Pulse all ingredients in a food processor until well-combined. Check the texture and make sure it stays combined when a small amount is pressed between your fingers. If not, add a little more maple syrup or a splash of water.

2. Roll the mixture into balls (5 larger ones, or 10 small ones) and store in the fridge.

Flavor Variations:

Chocolate chip: add ¼ cup chocolate chips

Pumpkin: add 2 Tb pumpkin puree, plus ¼ tsp pumpkin pie spice

Gingerbread: substitute 1 Tb of molasses for the maple syrup, add ⅛ tsp dried ginger, ⅛ tsp of cloves, and ¼ tsp of cinnamon. Optional: using a cookie cutter, shape them into gingerbread men, and let them masquerade as cookies at a holiday party

Lemon–blueberry: add the juice of ½ lemon, zest of ½ lemon, and ¼ cup dried blueberries

Cocoa–berry: add 1 Tb cocoa powder and 2 Tb dried berries

Orange–cranberry: add ½ tsp orange zest and a squeeze of fresh orange juice, along with ¼ cup dried cranberries

Peanut butter and jelly: use 2 Tb jelly/jam of choice instead of maple syrup

---

Snackable Smoothie (*P, C; P, F, C if you add nut butter or avocado*)

Customize your smoothie with extras. The possibilities are endless!

Makes 1 smoothie

1 cup water, coconut water, or milk of choice

1 scoop (21 g) protein powder (optional, but easy way to amp up nutrients and flavor)

½ cup frozen fruit of choice

½ banana or ¼ avocado

Extras:

1 cup greens (such as spinach or kale)

1 Tb coconut oil (will aid with nutrient absorption if you are adding greens)

1 tsp citrus zest

1 Tb sweetener (such as Stevia, unrefined sugar, honey, or dates)

1 Tb cocoa powder

1 Tb hemp seeds

1 Tb chocolate chips

1. Blend all ingredients in a high-speed blender and enjoy.

Additional tried-and-true favorites

- Mango, ½ banana, spinach, milk or fruit juice, and protein powder if desired

- Cherry–berry blend, ½ banana, avocado, cocoa powder, milk of choice, and protein powder

- Pineapple, spinach, shredded coconut, and milk of choice

- Mango, goji berry puree (soak and blend 2 Tb goji berries), orange juice, lime juice, and cayenne pepper (this is one of my all-time smoothie loves! Sweet and spicy)

- Strawberries, banana, milk of choice, lots of nut butter, and protein powder if desired (like a peanut butter and jelly sandwich)

- Banana, chocolate chips, spinach, fresh mint leaves, and milk of choice (tastes like a chocolate chip mint shake)

- Detox smoothie: one cup of water, one apple (leave the skin on!), one to two ribs of celery, a handful of fresh spinach, the juice of one lemon, 1 Tb of fat (coconut oil or chia seeds), and some mint or cilantro (for a spicier kick!)

Make ahead tip: To prep ahead, place all of your ingredients in the fridge in the blender, ready to go, and blend in the morning. If your blender does not detach from the lower mechanical part, place the ingredients in your to-go cup in the fridge. Plop into the blender in the morning, blend, and go.

Smoothie tips

- **Make sure to have a combination of liquid, fruit, texture (avocado, yogurt, and banana all help to yield a smooth texture), and mix-ins:** greens, veggies, superfoods, starches (uncooked oats, granola), fats (such as nuts or nut butters, hemp seeds, flax, chia), spices, and/or herbs. While it's tempting to want to add many ingredients, try to stay mindful of serving sizes and the overall nutritional impact of your smoothie.

- **Use frozen fruit instead of ice.** Ice waters down the smoothie and frozen fruit brings it down to the perfect temperature without sacrificing flavor.

- While blending, **blend at the "low-medium" speed until all of the ingredients are fully chopped** and combined (about two minutes). After this point, increase the speed all the way to high and blend for an additional minute. If you try to go to high speed right away, all of the fruit will migrate to the bottom and get stuck. If things aren't blending smoothly, add a little more liquid.

- One cool thing about enjoying smoothies as meals is that you can customize them to fit your nutritional needs. **I often suggest an extra smoothie to clients who are looking to gain weight.** It provides extra calories, without actually having to chew them. You just make the smoothie in the morning, leave it in the fridge, and make sure it's gone by the end of the day (in addition to the regular eats). If you're not looking to gain weight, **smoothies are a great choice for a quick and nutritious meal.** A half serving is a satisfying snack.

Perfect Protein Pancakes (*P, C*)

This is like the little black dress of high-protein breakfasts. It's always a great choice, and you can dress it up with fresh berries and pure maple syrup, or dress it down with a smear of nut butter and fold it up like a taco.

Makes 1 to 2 satisfying pancakes

    1½ scoops (31 g) protein powder (such as vanilla Sun Warrior)

    One egg white (not the carton kind)

    ¼ cup almond milk

    2 Tb whole grain flour (such as brown rice flour, spelt flour) or gluten-free flour mix (such as Bob's Red Mill Baking Mix)

    ¾ tsp baking powder

    ½ tsp cinnamon

    Pinch of nutmeg

    Pinch of sea salt

    ½ tsp vanilla

    Sweetener to taste (such as Stevia) (*optional*)

1. Heat a skillet to medium heat and spray lightly with olive oil or nonstick spray.

2. While the pan is heating up, in a small bowl, combine the protein powder, baking mix, baking powder, cinnamon, nutmeg, Stevia, and sea salt, and whisk to remove any lumps. Whisk in the egg white, almond milk, and vanilla.

3. Cook the pancake(s) for two to three minutes on each side, until golden brown. Serve topped with a drizzle of maple syrup, protein fluff, or jam. For an easy breakfast syrup, heat your favorite frozen berries on the stove at medium heat, and add 1 tsp of citrus zest and a little Stevia or sweetener of choice.

Tip: To make the pancakes vegan, use a flax egg instead of the egg white. Dissolve 1 Tb ground flax in 2 Tb of water or almond milk. Works like a charm!

Tip: If you'd like to double the recipe to freeze an extra batch, instead of using two egg whites, use the whole egg. The yolk is the best (and most nutritious) part!

Make ahead tip: To freeze extra pancakes, let them cool completely before placing flat in a freezer bag. I separate each cake with a small piece of parchment paper so they don't stick to one another. When you want to enjoy, put the frozen pancakes into the toaster.

Flax seeds

Flax seeds are best consumed in their ground state, as it's easier to absorb the nutrients and digest. They're a great source of healthy fats and wonderful in baked goods, sprinkled onto yogurts, oats, or in smoothies. Most grocery stores carry flax seed. If you're unable to find it already ground, you can easily grind the flax in a coffee grinder.

Turkey Lentil Muffins (*P, C*)

I originally made these turkey muffins for my daughter, who was then only a year old and starting to really enjoy feeding herself. They've remained a staple in our house because they freeze well and everyone enjoys them. These little protein muffins make a great snack dipped into mustard or ketchup; they're also wonderful as the "meatballs" in spaghetti, as a wrap filling, or as a salad topping.

Makes 12 muffins

> 2 cups cooked lentils
>
> 2 cups cooked quinoa
>
> ½ cup baby carrots
>
> 1 shallot
>
> 1 lb. extra lean ground turkey
>
> ½ cup barbecue (BBQ) sauce of choice plus additional for glaze (I use the Trader Joe's brand)
>
> ½ tsp dried sage
>
> ½ tsp garlic powder
>
> ½ tsp dried oregano

Sea salt to taste

Pepper to taste

1. Preheat the oven to 350° F. Coat a 12-cup muffin tin with nonstick spray or olive oil.

2. In a food processor, chop the carrots and shallot. Add the chopped veggies to a large bowl.

3. To this bowl, add the cooked quinoa, lentils, ground turkey, ½ cup BBQ sauce, sage, oregano, garlic powder, sea salt, and pepper. Stir to combine.

4. Transfer to the muffin tin and press down. Bake for 45 minutes. Top with more BBQ sauce to taste and bake for an additional 15 minutes.

5. Let the muffins cool completely before placing in the fridge (to help the BBQ sauce set better). When ready to serve, warm in the oven.

Tip: These are excellent scrambled into eggs or on top of a kale salad. For the salad, massage the torn leaves of one bunch of kale (yes, with your hands) for a few minutes, add a serving of your favorite salad dressing, then top with a crumbled turkey muffin.

Egg and Veggie Muffins (*P, F*)

I LOVE egg casseroles and dishes, but they're not realistic to make for an everyday, busy morning breakfast. By making a large batch of egg muffins or frittatas, you can freeze them and pop one in the microwave for a quick and hearty breakfast option.

Makes 10 mini frittatas

6 eggs

2 Tb milk of choice

1 Tb flour of choice (I use brown rice flour)

¾ cup shredded cheese (I use goat gouda)

1 cup chopped green veggies (broccoli, zucchini, spinach, or asparagus work well)

⅛ to ¼ tsp sea salt

¼ tsp garlic powder

⅛ tsp dried oregano

⅛ tsp dried thyme

Pinch of nutmeg

Red pepper flakes to taste (*optional*)

1. Preheat the oven to 350° F. Spray a 12-cup muffin tin with nonstick spray or olive oil.

2. In a large bowl, whisk the eggs and then stir in the remaining ingredients.

3. Pour into the muffin tins. If you use an ice cream scoop, it helps create muffins that are uniform size.

4. Bake for 20 to 22 minutes and let cool on a wire rack.

Make ahead tip: Freeze and reheat for an easy, protein-filled snack or with toast for a quick breakfast.

Chicken Spring or Nori Rolls (*P*)

This is one of those quick-and-easy lunches that rivals a restaurant meal (except for the fact that you had to make it for yourself ... and clean the dishes afterward) Bonus: they're fun party appetizers, too.

Makes 1 large serving

½ cup shredded rotisserie chicken (shrimp or tofu work well, too)

1 cup julienned veggies (cucumber and carrots are my favorites)

1 bunch leafy greens of choice, thinly sliced

1 package rice paper wraps or nori

Tamari or hot sauce, for dipping/drizzling

1. For spring rolls, have a shallow bowl of hot water ready. Work with one wrap at a time. Soak each wrap for 10 seconds. Roll a small amount of chicken, veggies, and greens in each wrap and seal tightly.

2. For nori rolls, no soaking is necessary. Roll a small amount of chicken, veggies, and greens in each wrap. Press and seal the edge with a damp paper towel.

3. Drizzle with a little tamari and/or hot sauce.

Cinnamon Quinoa Muffin Tops (*C*, *F*)

Makes 6 muffin tops

1 flax egg (1 Tb ground flax dissolved in 2 Tb milk of choice)

2 Tb cashew butter (almond butter would be good, too)

¼ cup pure maple syrup or agave

1 tsp vanilla

½ cup quinoa flakes (or shredded coconut flakes)

½ cup quinoa flour (or flour of choice)

½ tsp baking powder

½ tsp cinnamon

¼ tsp baking soda

Pinch of sea salt

Chocolate chips, chopped apples, chopped nuts, or dried fruit (*optional*)

1. Preheat the oven to 350° F and lightly grease a cookie sheet. In a mixing bowl, combine the flax egg, cashew butter, maple syrup, and vanilla until well combined.

2. In a separate large bowl, using a fork or whisk, combine the quinoa flakes, flour, cinnamon, baking soda, baking powder, and salt. If you're using mix-ins add dry mix-ins like chopped nuts or chocolate chips with the dry ingredients and the wet mix-ins like chopped apples and dried fruit to the cashew butter/syrup mixture.

3. With the mixer on low, add the flour mixture in batches to the wet mixture.

4. Using a melon ball scooper or tablespoon, scoop the mixture onto the cookie sheet, evenly spaced apart.

5. Bake for 10 minutes. Leave on the baking sheet for one additional minute, and transfer to a cooling rack to cool.

Tip: Enjoy topped with a smear of almond butter, a drizzle of melted butter, or solo. Freeze and reheat in the microwave as an easy, portable snack.

Banana Almond Muffins (*F, C*)

Makes 12 muffins

> 1 cup almond meal
>
> 1 cup brown rice or whole wheat flour
>
> 1 tsp cinnamon
>
> 1 tsp baking powder
>
> ⅛ tsp nutmeg
>
> Pinch of sea salt
>
> 3 ripe bananas, mashed
>
> 6 oz. (about ¾ cup) yogurt or canola oil
>
> 1 large egg or flax egg
>
> ¼ cup honey or liquid sweetener of choice
>
> 1 tsp vanilla extract
>
> 1 tsp molasses (*optional*)

1. Preheat the oven to 350° F. Grease a 12-cup muffin tin or line with muffin liners.
2. In a large bowl, combine the almond meal, flour, cinnamon, baking powder, nutmeg, and sea salt.
3. Add the bananas, egg, yogurt, honey, vanilla, and molasses and stir well.
4. Bake 25 to 30 minutes or until a toothpick inserted in the center comes out clean.
5. Try to let cool completely so you don't burn your mouth off. (This is where I fail.)

Tip: These are amazing topped with protein fluff or nut butter, crumbled onto oats, or by themselves.

Chocolate Protein Bars (*P, C*)

Makes 6 sizable squares (I have 2 or 3 for a snack)

> ⅓ cup sweet potato flesh from a large baked sweet potato (the canned stuff doesn't taste as good)

2 eggs plus 1 egg white

½ (3.5-oz) bar of chocolate

2 scoops protein powder of choice (I use vanilla Sun Warrior; chocolate would be awesome too)

⅓ cup brown rice flour

1 tsp vanilla

¼ tsp baking powder

Pinch of sea salt

Pinch of cinnamon

4 tsp (2 packs) of Stevia or sweetener of choice

1. Preheat oven to 350° F and spray an 8 x 8-inch baking dish with nonstick spray.

2. Melt the chocolate in a double boiler or microwave in a glass bowl, stirring at 30 second intervals.

3. Mix all of the ingredients in a large bowl. Pour mixture into the baking dish and smooth the top with a spatula.

4. Bake 20 minutes, or until toothpick comes out clean. Let cool completely and cut into six equal bars. Each bar can be wrapped in plastic and stored in the freezer in a large freezer bag.

Pumpkin Chocolate Chip Muffins (*F, C*)

Makes 6 muffins

⅓ cup pumpkin puree

2 Tb coconut oil

3 to 4 Tb of honey, to taste

3 eggs

1 tsp vanilla

½ cup almond meal

1 tsp baking powder

1 tsp baking soda

¼ to ½ cup mini chocolate chips

1 tsp pumpkin pie spice

Pinch of sea salt

1. Preheat the oven to 350° F. Spray a 12-cup muffin tin with nonstick spray or line with muffin cups.

2. In a large bowl, combine the pumpkin, coconut oil, honey, eggs, and vanilla. Set aside.

3. In a separate bowl, combine almond meal, baking powder, baking soda, chocolate chips, pumpkin pie spice, and sea salt.

4. Add the dry ingredients to the wet, and stir to combine.

5. Gently scoop the batter into the prepared muffin pan.

6. Bake 30 to 35 minutes, until golden brown and fluffy.

Eight easy snacks

Each week on Sunday, I like to make a fridge full of prepped food to enjoy during the week. Things get too crazy, and it's so much easier to grab something with little preparation to take with us wherever we're going. The first time I really stocked up the fridge, my husband thought we were having a party! Needless to say, he was pretty impressed with everything I'd made so quickly and also thankful when he had quick options to take to work. Any of my recipes can be prepared ahead for easy snacking throughout the week, but if you're really crunched for time, try these. These recipes are quickly made on the fly using minimal ingredients; for many of these, you may be surprised to have everything already on hand.

> **Veggies and hummus** *(veggies = N; hummus = C, F)*
> Take any crudités you enjoy and serve them with a few table-spoons of quick and easy homemade hummus. For the hummus, combine one 14 oz can of chickpeas (with half of the juice from the can), 1 Tb olive oil, two cloves of fresh garlic (or ½ tsp garlic powder), sea salt to taste, a pinch of cayenne, juice of half a lemon, and ½ tsp cumin in the food processor. It will be good in the fridge for a few days and is also fantastic on sandwiches, wraps, and in a salad with goat cheese and balsamic dressing.

Banana tortilla roll-up *(C, F, P)*
Make some protein fluff, or grab up a little nut or almond butter, smear it onto a tortilla, and place a banana in the tortilla. Roll it up like a burrito, and enjoy as a filling and energizing snack.

Protein yogurt *(P, F)*
Grab your favorite plain, no-sugar-added yogurt and top with berries, cinnamon, and a drizzle of honey.

Egg on toast with hot sauce *(P, F, C)*
Slice up a steamed or hard-boiled egg and enjoy with toast and hot sauce.

Tempeh slaw *(F, P)*
Mix ¼ block of tempeh with broccoli slaw and your favorite dressing.

Avocado salad *(F)*
Take ½ avocado and fill the pit hole with salsa or fresh pico de gallo. Eat plain or scooped onto ½ serving of tortilla chips.

Quinoa and caprese salad *(C, P, F)*
Mix ⅓ cup cooked quinoa with fresh basil, 1 oz of crumbled goat cheese, and halved cherry tomatoes. Season with garlic and sea salt.

Small baked sweet potato with goat cheese and chives *(C, P, F)*
Top a baked sweet potato (already baked on your prep day!) with soft goat cheese, a little sea salt, and chopped fresh chives.

Choosing pre- and postworkout fuel

There is a ton of debate out there regarding fasting before workouts, snacking beforehand, and ratio strategies. Here's my advice without turning it into a science experiment: If you're hungry before your workout, EAT! If you're not, you can skip it. For me, if I'm working out early, I prefer to do so on an empty stomach. If it's a later workout, I'll make sure to have a nice snack around an hour before so I'm not getting my sweat session with an uncomfortable food baby (that too-full-to-run or really do anything feeling).

In a 2011 study in the *International Journal of Sport Nutrition and Exercise Metabolism,* researchers compared the contrasting effects of eating and fasting preworkout. The group that ate enjoyed a classic Mediterranean breakfast before working out, while the fasting group did not eat until afterward. The group that ate had higher oxygen consumption postworkout than the fasting group, indicating an elevated metabolism, and also had a lower respiratory exchange ratio (RER). When your RER is high, your body is using a higher percentage of macronutrients from food (most carbs and fat) for energy. A lower RER occurs when the body is using stored fat in the body as its fuel source. I'll clank my fork to that! A little preworkout snack could actually HELP burn more fat. So if you're hungry—eat up, buttercup. Choose a snack that is low in fiber and has a nice ratio of carbs, fat, and protein.

Pre- and postworkout fuel! Some people like to have a small snack before a workout, while others feel like it's too heavy. Do what works best for you. If you choose to have a snack beforehand, make sure that it's a nice mix of carbohydrates and some protein with little fat and not too much fiber for easy digestion. Some good options: banana with almond butter, yogurt, small cup of granola with milk of choice, a serving of chicken or turkey on whole grain crackers, apple with goat cheese, small smoothie. Postworkout, be sure to enjoy some protein, carbs, and a little fat within 60 minutes of completing your workout. This combination will help facilitate muscle rebuilding and also replenish your glycogen stores. The ratio you should aim for immediately postworkout in terms of carbs:protein is about 4:1.

If you're training for an endurance event, you will also need to consume electrolytes and carbohydrates during sessions lasting longer than one hour. These can be homemade sports gels or sports drinks, dates, or purchased energy blocks. Try different types of fuel to find a type that will boost your energy without upsetting your stomach. Be sure to hydrate before, during, and after your workout.

Money-saving tips

1. **Shop around.** If you choose to go the organic route, it's advantageous to do some price hunting. When you buy organic, frozen is usually less expensive and is a great option for meat and berries. If organic isn't an option, conventional produce is better than no produce at all! Don't beat yourself up about it.

2. **Cook in bulk.** Making large batches of staple items (such as beans, grains, and bread) can be an ideal money-saving strategy. This is another reason why it's helpful to prep ahead, as you're more likely to have healthy options on hand (that is, fewer restaurant meals) and less likely to waste food that goes unprepped and thus unused.

3. **Check online for coupons.** Coupons can be especially helpful for more expensive groceries, including eggs, milk, nondairy milks, and snacks. Search your favorite brand online and pull up the coupon on your phone. It makes it easy to scan and save in the checkout line!

4. **Go for canned fish.** It's less expensive and just as nutrient-dense as the fresh version. Plus, if like me you live in the desert or some other similar area of the country and the closest ocean is pretty far away, all "fresh" seafood tends to be a little sketchy. Anchovies, sardines, canned salmon, and tuna are high-protein and healthy fat staples. Search for canned seafood that was fished with sustainable practices and make sure the can is BPA (Bisphenol A)-free. A quick scan of the label will let you know!

5. **Make your own pricey store-bought snacks at home.** Sure, it's a little bit more work, but far less expensive to make your own veggie chips, granola bars, and trail mix at home. See what's worth it for you! If the convenience factor is worth the price, by all means, enjoy, but if you're looking for easy ways to save some money, making your snacks at home is going to be kinder on the ol' wallet. Bonus: you can customize the ingredients to suit your personal preferences.

6. **Buy what you need.** While purchasing in bulk can be a saver in the long run, often you only need a tiny bit of certain ingredients. The bulk bins at most health food stores are a great option—if I'm baking a specialty recipe, I'll scope out the bins to measure

flour and nuts—and the local farmer's market is another good source. You can buy singles of fruits and veggies, instead of a large bag that you may not necessarily use.

7. **Go for frozen.** Frozen fruits and vegetables are often less expensive than fresh and are frozen at their peak of freshness. Some favorites: berries for smoothies, spinach for quiche, broccoli (a time-saver since I don't have to wash and cut an enormous head of broccoli), and certain herbs. Many grocery stores sell frozen trays of garlic and basil, which are a convenient flavor infusion.

8. **Grow your own.** If you have a green thumb—sadly, mine often kills plants with a single touch—it's very cost effective to grow your own produce or herbs. I usually have a harder time killing herbs than flowers, so we'll grow fresh basil, rosemary, cilantro, and parsley.

Chapter 8

HIIT Recipes

Here are some quick, healthy meals that can be made in 20 minutes or less, sans fancy kitchen equipment.

Breakfast

- Breakfast Cookie
- Baked Breakfast Cookie
- Berry Chia Pancakes
- Breakfast Cookie Dough Cereal
- Banana French Toast
- Sweet Potato Breakfast Casserole

The Breakfast Cookie *(C, F, P)*

This was my first original high-protein breakfast creation. I was looking for something with staying power that I could easily make the night before. Oats are one of my favorite breakfasts, but I found that I was often hungry a couple of hours later. The staying power of nut butter and protein powder, plus the fun option of flavor mix-ins helps to create a delicious and dessert-like breakfast treat. You can also make up to 5 breakfast cookies and store in the fridge to enjoy all week.

Makes 1 breakfast cookie

⅓ cup oats of choice (or raw buckwheat groats, ground into a flour)

1 Tb nut butter of choice (I'm on a sunflower seed butter kick, but peanut or almond butter are both great choices)

½ scoop (10 g) of protein powder (chocolate or vanilla, whatever you like! My current favorites are Jay Robb vanilla egg white protein or Sun Warrior vanilla)

2 to 4 Tb milk of choice (almond, hemp, rice, oat), depending on the texture you like

½ medium banana

Sweetener to taste (such as Stevia)

Pinch of cinnamon (optional)

Mix-ins: nuts, dried fruit, cocoa powder, cinnamon, chocolate chips

1. In a small bowl, add the oats, nut butter, and protein powder. Stir to combine and use the spoon to break up the nut butter until you have a nice crumbly mixture.

2. Add your milk of choice and mix until fully moistened.

3. Next, mash the ½ banana, add in, and stir well.

4. Now the fun part—pick the mix-ins! You can get creative with this. I've tried bananas, raisins, pumpkin, chocolate chips, ground espresso beans, and many other things; add anything you like. Stir in your mix-ins of choice and season (I enjoy a little Stevia and cinnamon).

5. Plop the mixture onto an appetizer-sized plate and with the back of your spoon flatten it into a round shape with equal thickness throughout.

6. Cover your cookie, either by storing it in a container or placing plastic wrap on top.

7. Put the cookie in the fridge overnight. It will harden slightly from the nut butter and the oats will soften from the milk.

8. Next morning, grab a spoon and enjoy!

Baked Breakfast Cookie *(C, F, P)*

Over the years that many of my readers tried (and loved!) the original breakfast cookie, I found that some people weren't crazy about the texture. Some didn't really like the overnight oats-esque texture, and some people are allergic to (or just despise) bananas. This version is just as nutrient-dense, but really is like a cookie. Cookies for breakfast—wahoo!

Makes 8 cookies

> 2 cups oats
>
> 2 scoops vanilla protein powder
>
> 1 tsp baking soda
>
> ¼ tsp cinnamon
>
> Pinch sea salt
>
> 1 (4-oz) container of applesauce
>
> 1 egg
>
> ½ tsp vanilla
>
> 1 pack (2 tsp) Stevia (or sweetener to taste)
>
> ½ cup nut butter of choice
>
> ¼ to ½ cup chocolate chips, dried fruit, or any mix-ins you love.
>   *If you're not using chocolate chips, I'd be sure to add in some brown sugar or something similar, since the chocolate adds a nice amount of sweetness.

1. Preheat the oven to 350° F and spray a large cookie sheet with olive oil or nonstick spray.

2. Mix the oats, protein powder, baking soda, cinnamon, sea salt, and any mix-ins in a large bowl. Next, add the egg, applesauce, and sweetener. Mix well.

3. Using your hands (it helps to wet them a little as the dough is sticky!), shape the dough into eight large cookies and place on the greased baking sheet.

4. Bake 10 to 12 minutes. Let cool on the baking sheet and store in the fridge (eat within three days) or in the freezer to reheat, and enjoy.

Berry Chia Pancakes *(C, F, P)*

One of my favorite things to cook for breakfast is pancakes, but during a busy week they're a little too labor-intensive. Instead, I'll make a large batch during the weekend. After they cook, I'll separate them with sheets of parchment paper and place in a ziplock bag in the freezer. All I have to do is put the pancake in the toaster and "pop!" breakfast is served. My daughter loves these berry chia pancakes with fresh fruit, syrup, and an egg on the side.

Makes about 8 pancakes

> 1 cup flour of choice (brown rice flour is gluten free and works beautifully with this recipe)
>
> 1 tsp baking powder
>
> Pinch of sea salt
>
> ½ medium banana
>
> 1 egg
>
> 1 tsp chia seeds
>
> ½ cup fresh or thawed frozen berries
>
> ⅔ cup milk of choice (I use almond)
>
> 1 tsp vanilla

1. Heat a sauté pan on low while you make the mix.
2. In a large bowl, whisk together the flour, baking powder, and salt.
3. On a small plate, mash the banana with the chia seeds.
4. Plop the banana mixture into the dry mixture, add the egg, milk, and vanilla. Whisk well.
5. Add a little coconut oil or butter to your pan then, using an ice cream scoop or ¼ cup measure, scoop your first pancake into the pan.
6. Cook for one to two minutes on the first side, add a few berries, and flip.
7. Cook the second side until browned to perfection, about 30 seconds to 1 minute. And, if you're like us, eat as you cook.

Chia seeds

Chia seeds are from the desert plant *Salvia hispanica*, and yes, they are the seeds used to create the infamous chia pet "hair." They're a filling, hydrating addition to meals and snacks and also yield a gelatinous texture when soaked in liquid. You can find chia seeds online and at health food stores. Word to the wise: keep some floss with ya.

Breakfast Cookie Dough Cereal *(C, F, P)*

This recipe was created when I really wanted a breakfast cookie but lacked the foresight to make one the night before. I decided to use the same ingredients but crumble them into a bowl to yield a cookie dough-esque cereal. A new breakfast favorite was born!

Makes 1 satisfying bowl

⅓ to ½ cup oats (depending on how hungry you are)

½ scoop (11 g) protein powder of choice

1 Tb nut butter of choice (cashew, almond, peanut, and sunflower seed butter all work nicely)

1 cup milk of choice

Sweetener of choice (such as Stevia)

½ tsp vanilla

Pinch of cinnamon

Pinch of sea salt

Toppings of choice! Fresh fruit, berries, nuts, hemp seeds, the possibilities are endless.

1. In a bowl, add the oats, protein powder, cinnamon, sea salt, sweetener, and vanilla.

2. Mix well to combine. Add your favorite nut butter, and using a spoon, break up and stir until mixture resembles crumbly cookie dough.

3. Top with at least 1 cup milk of choice, and then add fun toppings.

4. Grab a spoon and enjoy!

Banana French Toast *(C, F, P)*

You'd never believe that this vegan twist on French toast is completely egg free! Not only does that banana help to provide a light fluffy texture, it also yields a crisp texture and light sweetness. These are an ideal make-ahead breakfast.

Makes 1 serving

1 mashed banana

½ scoop (about 10 g) of your favorite protein powder (*optional*)

2 Tb milk of choice

1 Tb ground flax

¼ tsp vanilla

Pinch of cinnamon

2 slices of your favorite bread

Coconut oil or butter for cooking

Maple syrup and chopped fresh fruit for serving

1. In a bowl, combine the banana, milk, flax, vanilla, cinnamon, and protein powder if you decide to use it. Heat a small pan to medium-low.

2. Dip the bread in the banana (the faux egg) mixture and flip over to coat well.

3. Add a little butter or coconut oil to the pan and add the first slice to the pan. Cook for two to three minutes per side until golden brown. Repeat with the other slice.

4. Serve with pure maple syrup and fresh berries.

Make Ahead Tip: These freeze extremely well, so if you have some bananas on their last leg, it's a great alternative to banana bread. When you want to reheat, just put each piece in the toaster.

Flavor Variations: Try topping with peanut butter and jelly, or fresh berries and a sprinkle of chocolate chips. Protein fluff also makes a killer French toast and pancake topping!

Sweet Potato Breakfast Casserole *(C, F, P)*

This is a fiesta in a casserole dish. It has all of the textures and flavor combos covered, plus it's an ideal balance of protein, healthy fats, and smart carbs. Try leftovers atop salad greens for lunch, too!

Makes 8 servings

   8 eggs

   ½ cup almond milk

   ½ tsp smoked paprika

   ½ tsp garlic powder

   1 bag of fresh spinach, lightly sautéed to wilt

   ½ cup of your favorite cheese

   2 large baked sweet potatoes, sliced

   1. Preheat the oven to 350° F and spray a standard casserole dish with nonstick spray.
   2. Add the sweet potato slices to the bottom of the dish. Top with cheese and sautéed spinach.
   3. Whisk the eggs, milk, and seasonings in a bowl and pour the egg mixture on top of the sweet potatoes, cheese, and spinach.
   4. Bake for 30 minutes until golden brown and set.

Tip: Cut into portion-sized pieces, and freeze any leftovers to enjoy with a large salad for lunch later during the week!

Lunch
   - Cashew Avocado Salad
   - Quinoa Power Salad
   - Deconstructed Sushi Salad

- Thai Shredded Chicken Lettuce Wraps

- Eggplant Pizza

- Zucchini Pizza

- Kale Slaw with Ginger Miso Dressing

- Marinara Veggie Bake

- Quinoa Bake

Cashew Avocado Salad *(F)*

This is a very simple salad, but the flavors combine extremely well! It's my own at-home version of a beloved salad from Renee's Organic Oven in Tucson.

Makes 1 large salad

2 cups of your favorite salad greens (spinach and arugula work extremely well in this salad)

½ avocado, sliced

¼ cup cashews

1 Tb fresh chives, chopped

Red wine vinegar

Olive oil

Sea salt to taste

Pepper to taste

1. In a large bowl, add the lettuce, avocado, cashews, and chives.

2. Toss well to combine.

3. Drizzle with a little vinegar and olive oil, then top with a sprinkle of salt and pepper.

Make Ahead Tip: Combine the lettuce and chives in a to-go container, top with ½ avocado, and drizzle some fresh lime or lemon on top to prevent browning. Seal the container and place in the fridge; on the counter, prep a little baggie of cashews and a small container with red wine vinegar, olive oil, salt, and pepper. When you're ready to eat the next day, add the cashews and dressing, toss, and feast!

Quinoa Power Salad *(C, P, F)*

This salad is a fantastic dose of protein, antioxidants, and healthy fats. It's a wonderful balanced meal for packed lunches or a quick dinner. Since there are so many flavors and textures in this salad, a simple seasoning goes a long way.

Makes 4 satisfying servings

    2 cups cooked quinoa

    1 cup dried fruit of choice (cranberries and cherries are particularly lovely; just make sure to purchase the unsweetened variety)

    1 large avocado, sliced

    1 cup salad greens of choice, shredded

    ½ cup chopped almonds

    1 cup garbanzo beans

    2 Tb olive oil

    Juice of ½ lemon

    Pinch of garlic powder

    Sea salt to taste

    Pepper to taste

1. In a large bowl, toss the salad greens, quinoa, fruit, avocado, almonds, and beans until well-mixed.

2. Drizzle with a little olive oil, season liberally with garlic powder, salt, and pepper, and then add a squeeze of lemon juice. Enjoy!

Make Ahead Tip: Cook the quinoa in your Sunday prep. Combine all of the salad ingredients, except the avocado. Store covered in the fridge for three to five days. This is also fantastic split up into Mason jars to take to work. When you're ready to eat, add the avocado, oil, lemon juice, and seasonings. Enjoy!

Deconstructed Sushi Salad *(C, F, P)*

This salad combines classic sushi flavors into a delightful salad bowl. Feel free to customize with your protein and veggie options!

Makes 1 large salad

½ cup of your favorite sushi grain (quinoa and brown rice are lovely; you could also use steamed chopped cauliflower as a grain-free option)

½ cup chopped salad greens

4 oz smoked salmon, tuna, or sliced tempeh

Chopped veggies, such as cucumber, carrots, bell pepper

1 sheet of nori, chopped or torn (found in the Asian section of most grocery stores)

Tamari or soy sauce

Pinch of garlic powder

Pinch of cayenne *(optional)*

Sriracha *(optional, but highly recommended)*

1. In a large bowl, add your grain of choice, salad greens, veggies, and salmon.

2. Top with the chopped nori (which I really prefer to tear into bite-sized pieces with my hands like a sushi barbarian) and drizzle lightly with tamari or soy sauce.

3. Toss to combine and season with cayenne and a sprinkle of garlic powder.

Make Ahead Tip: Combine the greens, grains (which should already be prepped and ready to go for the week), salmon, and chopped veggies (also prepped) in your to-go container. Season with cayenne and garlic powder. Store the container in the fridge for the next morning. Place the chopped nori in a baggie on the counter (so it doesn't get soggy) and a little pack of tamari or soy sauce (or you can take the bottle with you). When you're ready to enjoy your sushi salad, add the nori and tamari, toss, and eat! This is also fantastic with a drizzle of sriracha if you're a spicy fanatic like myself.

Thai Shredded Chicken Lettuce Wraps *(P, F)*

Chicken lettuce wraps are a high-protein dinner or lunch option. For these, the creamy and slightly spicy dressing takes them over the top. Bonus: they make fun party appetizers, too.

Makes 1 large serving

  2 Tb nut butter of choice (almond and peanut butter are both great)

  1 Tb milk of choice

  1 tsp tamari

  ½ tsp honey

  ¼ teaspoon garlic powder

  Sea salt to taste

  Pepper to taste

  4 large leaves romaine lettuce

  1 cup shredded chicken

  1 sliced bell pepper

  Sliced pineapple

  1 Tb fresh mint

  1 Tb fresh cilantro

1. In a small bowl combine the nut butter, milk, tamari, honey, garlic powder, salt, and pepper.
2. Add the chicken and toss to coat.
3. Spoon the mixture onto the pieces of romaine. Top with bell pepper, pineapple, cilantro, and mint.
4. Roll up and eat like a taco!

Eggplant Pizza *(F)*

I first fell in love with eggplant pizzas during my forays into low-carb eating. Although I happily embrace healthy carbs now, I still enjoy the meaty texture and burst of nutrition from using a sliced eggplant as the "crust." These delicious pizzas make a wonderful vegetarian dinner option and are even better the next day.

Makes 2 large servings. (Save the leftovers for dinner the next day!)

    1 eggplant, sliced into 1-inch rounds

    Olive oil or ghee

    Sea salt to taste

    Pepper to taste

    Toppings of choice (I use hummus, goat cheese, tomatoes, bell pepper, and fresh basil; sprouted tofu and grilled chicken are fantastic protein options)

1. Preheat the oven to 350° F and grease a cookie sheet with nonstick spray.

2. Place the eggplant rounds on the cookie sheet and top with olive oil or ghee, salt, and pepper.

3. Bake for 20 minutes until soft, but not mushy.

4. Add your favorite toppings. You can use marinara or hummus for the sauce, and have fun adding your favorite vegetable toppings. Fresh herbs such as basil should go on the pizzas just before serving. Get creative!

5. Bake for 10 additional minutes until everything is heated through.

6. Garnish with chopped fresh herbs and serve.

Tip: Remember that eggplants can soak up a lot of fat easily. Use an olive oil sprayer or nonstick spray if you are watching your fat intake.

Make Ahead Tip: Roast the eggplant rounds along with your favorite veggies to last the week. When you feel like eggplant pizza, grab a few rounds, top with your favorite toppings, heat (in the oven or in the microwave), and eat.

Zucchini Pizza *(P, F)*

This recipe is one of my favorite ways to get our daughter to eat an extra serving of green veggies. The zucchini gives the pizzas a bright color, and the savory pancake-like crust is a great vehicle for your favorite pizza toppings.

Makes 2 pizzas

      1 large zucchini

      ½ cup almond meal

      1 heaping Tb flax meal

      1 egg

      ½ tsp garlic powder

      ½ tsp dried oregano

      ½ tsp dried rosemary

      ¼ tsp sea salt

      ⅛ tsp pepper

      Butter or olive oil for pan

      Pizza toppings of choice

1. Grate the zucchini, place shreds in a small bowl, and sprinkle with sea salt. Let this sit while you prepare the rest of the ingredients. Drain and squeeze out any excess liquid.

2. Heat a skillet on medium-low while you mix the zucchini, almond meal, flax meal, egg, garlic powder, organo, rosemary, salt, and pepper in a large bowl.

3. Add a little butter or oil to the pan, and half of the batter to make a large pancake-type shape.

4. Cook for three minutes on each side, or until the batter is browned and cooked thoroughly.

5. Top with pizza toppings of choice, or use as bread for a sandwich!

Kale Slaw with Ginger Miso Dressing *(F, P)*

Kale salads are one of my lunchtime staples, and I decided to switch up the usual massaged kale salad with a bright and savory ginger miso dressing. The miso also adds some bonus probiotics to a nutritious and satisfying salad.

Makes 2–3 servings

  2 cups kale, washed, ribs removed, and torn into bite-sized pieces

  2 large carrots, peeled and shredded

  1 cucumber, peeled, seeded, and chopped (if using an English cucumber, just wash and dice)

  ½ cup grape tomatoes, halved

  Protein of choice (optional) (seafood, chicken, and tempeh are all wonderful options)

For dressing

  2 Tb chickpea miso, or miso paste of choice (found in the cold section of health food stores. Can't find it? Use 2 Tb soy sauce or tamari instead!)

  2 Tb rice vinegar

  1 heaping Tb honey

  2 garlic cloves, finely minced

  ½ tsp fresh minced ginger

  1 tsp sesame oil

  2 tsp olive oil

  Juice of ½ lime

  1. Place the kale, carrots, cucumber, and tomatoes in a large bowl.
  2. Whisk all of the dressing ingredients together in a separate bowl.
  3. Pour the desired amount of dressing on top of the salad, along with any protein you'd like to include. A little dressing

goes a long way! It's thick and savory. If you prefer a thinner dressing, add more oil and/or vinegar.

Make Ahead Tip: The most time-intense portion of this recipe (and most recipes in general) is the chopping. If you have your veggies washed and chopped in the beginning of the week, you can also make your dressing in advance to enjoy. This way, when you want a kale salad, you just pour in your ingredients, add the dressing, and enjoy! Save any extra dressing to use throughout the week, or double it to use as a marinade for your weekly protein.

Marinara Veggie Bake *(F)*

This veggie bake is the epitome of comfort food, but has a surprisingly low caloric toll. You can add any veggies you love!

Makes 4 large servings

  1 (28-oz) can of San Marzano whole peeled tomatoes, drained

  1 medium yellow onion, chopped

  2 cloves garlic, minced

  2 bell peppers, sliced into thick strips

  1 (8-oz) container Portobello mushrooms, washed and sliced

  2 zucchini or summer squash, sliced

  4 oz cheese of choice (goat cheese is my personal fave)

  2 Tb balsamic vinegar

  1 Tb of olive oil

  Pinch of sugar

  Sea salt to taste

  Pepper to taste

  Fresh basil, for garnish

1. Preheat the oven to 375° F.
2. In a large roasting dish, add all of the above ingredients, breaking the tomatoes up with a wooden spoon.

3. Season with salt and pepper, and crumble the cheese on top.

4. Cover with foil and bake for 20 minutes. Top with fresh basil and serve with your favorite Paleo or whole-grain bread for dipping.

Make Ahead Tip: Make this as part of your Sunday prep. Portion into separate containers to heat and enjoy throughout the week. To boost up the protein, add grilled chicken, sliced tempeh, or garbanzo beans. You can also serve this on top of spinach to increase satiety power.

Quinoa Bake *(C, P, F)*

This broccoli and mushroom quinoa casserole is a warm and hearty dinner option. Like most casseroles, it tastes even better the next day! This is a great Sunday prep option to heat for lunches and dinner throughout the week.

Makes 2 servings

½ cup quinoa, rinsed

1½ cups chicken or vegetable broth

1 medium yellow onion, chopped

2 bell peppers, chopped

1 (6- to 8-oz) container mushrooms, washed and sliced

1½ cups broccoli florets, chopped

2 Tb nutritional yeast

4 oz crumbled goat cheese

1 tsp dry mustard powder

1 tsp dried oregano

1 tsp dried thyme

¼ tsp sea salt

⅛ tsp pepper

Lemon slices for serving

Chopped fresh parsley for garnish

1. Preheat the oven to 350° F.

2. Combine all ingredients in a large casserole dish.

3. Bake for 30 minutes, until quinoa is cooked and fluffy.

4. Squeeze fresh lemon juice on top, and add chopped parsley for garnish.

Make Ahead Tip: Have all of your veggies chopped and ready to go. You can also make this dish as part of your Sunday prep. The leftovers are fabulous lunch options!

Dinner

- Orange Honey Salmon

- Chicken and Sweet Potato Burgers

- Jalepeno Turkey Burgers

- Butternut Squash Mac N' Cheesze

- Slow Cooker Bean-Free Chili

- Slow Cooker Cashew Chicken

- Slow Cooker Sweet Potato and Black Bean Chili

- Southwestern Crock-Pot Chicken

- Channa Masala

- Stuffed Chicken

- Fish Tacos with Creamy Lime-Chili Sauce

- Quinoa Sushi

- Warm Tempeh Salad with Mustard Vinaigrette

Orange Honey Salmon *(P, F)*

This is one of the very first "fancy" meals I learned to cook. My chef uncle, who was living in Key West at the time, gave me the instructions via phone—I was trying to impress a certain Pilot. Needless to say, the salmon came out beautifully; it's been one of our staple dinners ever since.

Makes 2 servings

  Zest of 1 orange

  Juice of 1 orange

  1 orange, sliced into rounds

  Small coin of ginger, grated

  3 cloves garlic, minced

  2 Tb tamari

  1 tsp honey

  2 (4-oz) filets wild salmon

  Sea salt to taste

  Pepper to taste

1. In a large bag, combine the orange zest, juice, and slices with ginger, garlic, tamari, and honey.

2. Salt and pepper the salmon well, and add to the bag. Seal and refrigerate for 20 minutes, or overnight.

3. When ready to cook, grease a baking dish and preheat the oven to 375° F. Preheat a large skillet to high and add a drizzle of olive oil. When the olive oil begins to dance and sizzle, add the salmon, skin side up (if you're using salmon with skin). Pan sear for 30 seconds to one minute, until the top layer is beautifully browned.

4. Using a spatula, remove the salmon from the pan, and flip to add to the baking dish (so the skin side is now down, and the golden pan-seared side is up). Top with the orange slices and drizzle a little extra marinade on top.

5. Cook for 10 to 15 minutes, or until it flakes easily with a fork.

Tip: If you're cooking for one, save the extra salmon filet to enjoy on whole grain toast with an egg the next day.

Chicken and Sweet Potato Burgers *(P, C)*

These are one of my favorite weekly staple recipes. The sweet potatoes add an unexpected smooth texture, along with slight sweetness and a boost of nutrients. It's a great way to amp up the usual protein burgers!

Makes 4 burgers

> 1 lb. of ground organic chicken
>
> Flesh of one medium-size baked sweet potato (about 3.5 oz)
>
> 2 Tb fresh parsley, chopped
>
> 2 garlic cloves, minced
>
> 1 tsp smoked paprika
>
> Sea salt to taste
>
> Pepper to taste

1. Preheat the oven to 375° F. Spray a standard cookie sheet with olive oil or nonstick spray.
2. In a large bowl, combine all of the ingredients and shape the mixture into four equal burger patties.
3. Bake for 20 minutes.

Tip: These burgers are especially wonderful on top of a fresh green salad, in a wrap, or scrambled with some eggs and veggies.

Make Ahead Tip: Make these burgers during your Sunday prep. Allow the burgers to cool to room temperature before storing in the fridge. Separate each burger using a small piece of parchment paper before freezing or storing in the fridge. When you're ready to enjoy, either microwave for a couple of minutes or throw on a greased skillet (medium heat) for three to five minutes per side.

Jalapeno Turkey Burgers *(P)*

This is the Pilot's top-secret recipe (!) and he is quite the burger king.

Makes 4 burgers

> 1 lb. lean ground turkey
>
> 1 Tb Worcestershire sauce

½ cup pickled jalapenos, chopped

1 small onion, finely diced

2 cloves garlic, minced

Pure maple syrup, drizzle to taste

Sea salt to taste

Pepper to taste

1. Preheat the grill.
2. While the grill is heating, combine all of the burger ingredients in a large bowl. Equally divide and shape into four patties.
3. Cook the burgers on the grill, flipping once halfway through.

Tip: Save the extra burgers (if there are any!), chop, and add to your salad the next day. It's a lean way to get in an extra 20 plus grams of protein.

Butternut Squash Mac n' Cheeze *(C, F, P)*

You'll never guess that this is a dairy-free version of the classic fave. The nutritional yeast in this recipe yields a gloriously cheesy flavor, and the cashews provide a creamy texture. Make this to impress your favorite vegetarian friend, or enjoy as part of a Meatless Monday.

Makes 4 servings

1 shallot, finely minced

1 cup raw cashews, soaked in water for at least 1 hour

1 cup steamed butternut squash

1 cup almond milk (or milk of choice)

½ cup nutritional yeast

1 tsp dried mustard powder

¼ tsp sea salt

Pepper to taste

Smoked paprika to taste

1 lb. of your favorite penne pasta (I love brown rice and quinoa pasta)

Spinach, to serve (*optional*)

1. Chop and sauté the shallot in a little butter or olive oil for about five minutes.

2. Add the shallot to a high-speed blender, along with the cashews, butternut squash, milk, nutritional yeast, mustard powder, sea salt, pepper, and paprika.

3. Blend until smooth and creamy. Taste and adjust seasonings as needed.

4. In the meantime, boil your pasta noodles as recommended on the box. If you're using gluten-free noodles, be careful not to overcook them. They will turn into a gooey, sticky mess. Season the pasta water generously with sea salt.

5. When the noodles are finished cooking, drain them over the sink and rinse with cold water. Add the cheesy sauce to the pot, and then the noodles, stirring over low heat.

6. Serve atop a bed of spinach for a delicious and nutrient-packed meal!

Slow Cooker Bean-Free Chili *(P)*

This variation on the classic recipe skips the beans. Over time, I've made quite a few chili variations depending on what we've had on hand. For one occasion, we didn't have any beans, and I figured it would be a great chance to use up as many veggies as possible. This chili is especially delicious with sliced avocado and a squeeze of lime juice.

Makes 4 large servings

1 lb. organic chicken or turkey sausage, chopped

2 zucchini, sliced

1 (28-oz) can whole, peeled tomatoes, drained

4 sweet potatoes, peeled and diced

2 red bell peppers, chopped

2 cups chicken broth

½ to 1 cup water

1 tsp chili powder

2 cloves of garlic, minced

1 tsp smoked paprika

Sea salt to taste

Pepper to taste

Scallions, sliced, to serve

Fresh parsley, chopped, to serve

1. Combine sausage, zucchini, tomatoes, sweet potatoes, bell peppers, broth, water, chili powder, garlic, paprika, salt, and pepper in the bowl of the slow cooker. Using the back of a wooden spoon, break up the tomatoes into smaller pieces.

2. Cook on high three to four hours, or on low for four to six hours, adding water for additional liquid if needed. Make sure that you have enough liquid to cover the vegetables, and more if you prefer more of a soup texture. Serve topped with scallions or parsley.

Make Ahead Tip: This chili freezes extremely well! You could make an entire batch and freeze in servings to enjoy later, or place all ingredients in a large freezer bag and store in the freezer. When you want to enjoy the chili the next day, allow to thaw overnight in the fridge and place in the slow cooker in the morning.

Slow Cooker Cashew Chicken (P, F)

I love takeout, but don't love the fact that I usually can't squeeze my rings onto my hands the next day from all of the sodium. When you make it at home, you can control the salt content, and also can make sure you're using fresh, whole ingredients. Here's one of my favorite at-home takeout recipes.

Makes 6 servings

2 lb. chicken breasts or thighs, washed, patted dry, and cut into bite-sized pieces

½ tsp salt

¼ tsp pepper

¼ tsp garlic powder

1½ cups chicken broth

¼ cup tamari

2 Tb rice vinegar

2 Tb tomato paste

1 Tb honey

2 garlic cloves, minced

½ tsp dried ginger

½ cup chopped cashews

Scallions, sliced, to serve

Sesame seeds, to serve

Cooked rice, quinoa, or sautéed zucchini, to serve. I usually do ½ cup rice/quinoa or a whole zucchini per person.

1. Place the chicken breasts in the slow cooker. Season liberally with salt, pepper, and garlic power.

2. Add the chicken broth and cook on low for three to four hours.

3. When the chicken is finished cooking, shred the meat. Next, make your sauce in a medium bowl by combining the tamari, rice vinegar, tomato paste, honey, garlic, and dried ginger. Whisk well to combine.

4. Pour the sauce over the chicken, stir to coat, and top with chopped cashews.

5. Serve over rice, sautéed zucchini, or cooked quinoa. Top with sliced scallions or a sprinkle of sesame seeds.

Tip: This chicken is also a fantastic lettuce wrap filling. Wash some stalks of romaine and fill with the mixture for a savory lunch option!

Slow Cooker Sweet Potato and Black Bean Chili *(C, P)*

This is one of the first recipes I made for the blog, and is one that I've come back to quite a few times. Even when I don't measure the ingredients exactly, it still yields a comforting, savory, and mildly sweet meal. It freezes well, and is a great dinner option to make for vegetarian friends or family.

Makes 4 large servings

    2 medium-size sweet potatoes, peeled and diced

    1 small sweet onion, diced

    1 red bell pepper, seeded and diced

    1 (14-oz) can of fire roasted tomatoes, drained

    1 (14-oz) can black beans, washed and drained

    1½ cups vegetable broth

    3 garlic cloves minced

    1 tsp cumin

    1 tsp paprika or smoked paprika

    ½ tsp sea salt

    Pinch of cayenne

    1 lime, quartered, for serving

    Greek yogurt, for serving

    Fresh cilantro, for serving

1. Spray a standard slow cooker dish with nonstick spray.
2. Add the sweet potato, onion, bell pepper, tomatoes, black beans, broth, garlic, cumin, paprika, salt, and cayenne to the slow cooker. Stir to combine and cook on low for four to six hours.
3. Squeeze lime juice before serving, and garnish with dollops of Greek yogurt and/or chopped, fresh cilantro.

Store covered in the fridge for up to five days. This chili also freezes extremely well, if you want to separate into servings and freeze for later.

Southwestern Crock-Pot Chicken *(P)*

This is my standard prep-ahead meal. The chicken tastes fantastic with a favorite salsa stirred in, and for serving suggestions, the possibilities are endless. You can enjoy this chicken on a bed of sautéed zucchini, steamed broccoli, sweet potato, in a sandwich, wrap, salad … anything! Hope you enjoy.

Makes 2–4 large servings, depending on how many chicken breasts you use

  2–4 medium-size chicken breasts

  1–1⅓ cups chicken broth

  1 tsp oregano

  1 tsp cumin

  Salt and pepper to taste

  ½ cup salsa, optional

1. Place chicken breasts and seasonings into the slow cooker. Fill with chicken broth halfway up the sides of the chicken (1½–2 cups).

2. Cook on high for three to four hours, or on low for four to six hours, making sure to keep enough liquid in the container— don't be afraid to add more water or broth as needed.

3. When the chicken is thoroughly cooked, shred the meat and stir in one jar of your favorite salsa. This is wonderful in breakfast burritos, on top of salads, or in quesadillas with your favorite cheese, some lettuce, and salsa.

Channa Masala *(C, P)*

When we were stationed in Valdosta, I always looked forward to Indian Food Wednesday. After teaching spin and Zumba, my friends and I would often head to the local Indian restaurant for a late night of sharing dishes and naan. When I became brave enough to attempt Indian cuisine at home, I went with channa masala, which is a beloved vegetarian dish. It's spicy, bold, and perfect to scoop up with some toasted naan bread.

Makes 6 large servings

  1 sweet onion, chopped

  2 cloves of garlic

  ½ tsp minced fresh ginger

1 tsp cumin

1 tsp turmeric

½ tsp ground coriander

½ tsp garam masala

¼ tsp cayenne (*optional*)

¼ to ½ tsp of sea salt

⅛ tsp pepper

2 (14- to 16-oz) cans of garbanzo beans, rinsed and drained

1 (28-oz) can of peeled tomatoes

Juice of one lemon

Steamed vegetables, brown rice, or quinoa, to serve

1. In a large sauté pan, cook the onions, garlic, and ginger on medium heat in a little olive oil or butter until translucent.

2. Next, add the spices (cumin, turmeric, coriander, garam masala, cayenne, salt, and pepper) and use a wooden spoon to stir and coat the onion/garlic mixture.

3. Add in the chickpeas and tomatoes, reducing the heat to low. Use a spoon or spatula to break up the tomatoes into the mixture. Allow to cook on low for 10 minutes.

4. Remove from the stove and serve over steamed vegetables, brown rice, or quinoa.

Tip: This mixture freezes extremely well! It's also delicious cooked in the slow cooker. I add a bunch of vegetables (chopped zucchini, squash, carrots) to the mixture and add the beans right before serving (since they're fully cooked and turn into mush when cooked for too long). Set it on low for four hours and enjoy an Indian-spiced veggie dinner.

Stuffed Chicken *(P, F)*

This is my go-to recipe when I want something quick, protein-packed, delicious, and surprisingly fancypants. I commonly make this one to take over when a friend has a baby, since it's a satisfying and visually appealing meal ... much better than the chocolate-covered acai berries I constantly shoved in my face during Livi's newborn days.

Makes 4 servings (if you're cooking for yourself, you can halve this recipe or make all four chicken breasts to add to salads, omelets, and wraps during the week)

> 4 medium-size chicken breasts
>
> 4 oz goat cheese (plain or herbed)
>
> ¼ cup fresh basil, chiffonade (cut into thin strips)
>
> 4 sundried tomatoes in olive oil, drained
>
> 2 lemons (one halved, one sliced)
>
> 2 cloves garlic, minced
>
> 1 tsp dried oregano
>
> Sea salt to taste
>
> Pepper to taste

1. Preheat the oven to 375° F. Spray a standard glass baking dish with nonstick spray or olive oil.

2. Pat the chicken dry, and using a sharp knife, create a horizontal cut two-thirds of the way across each chicken breast.

3. Add 1 oz of goat cheese, 1 Tb of fresh basil, and 1 tsp of sundried tomatoes to each chicken breast in the "pocket" you created, and place the top part of the chicken breast firmly down to secure. Place into your baking dish.

4. Top each chicken breast with salt and pepper, oregano, garlic, and one to two slices of fresh lemon. Place the halved lemon in the baking dish, too.

5. Bake for 15 to 20 minutes, until the chicken is cooked through and the juices run clear. (My cheater tip: I ALWAYS use a meat thermometer, or I'd cook meats until they're a white, chewy eraser. The general recommendation for chicken to be fully cooked is 165° F.)

6. Squeeze the juice from the roasted halved lemon onto the chicken before serving.

Fish Tacos with Creamy Lime-Chili Sauce *(P, F, C)*

Taco Tuesday! Or any day that ends with "y." This is a quick-and-easy dinner option, which pleases pretty much everyone. Make sure to load up with your favorite toppings, without skimping on the chili-lime sauce. You can also enjoy the fish taco salad-style on a bed of lettuce.

Makes 4 servings

1 lb. fish of choice (salmon, tilapia, and halibut all work beautifully)

½ tsp chili powder

½ tsp oregano

¼ tsp salt

⅛ tsp pepper

2 limes: 1 zested and juiced, 1 reserved

Hot sauce to taste

1 (6-oz) container of Greek yogurt

Corn or brown rice tortillas

Shredded lettuce

Avocado

Salsa

Black beans

Lime wedges, to serve

1. Preheat the oven to 375° F. Prepare your fish by placing it in a greased baking dish. Season with the chili powder, oregano, salt, pepper, lime zest, and juice.

2. Bake for 10 to 12 minutes, until easily flaked with a fork.

3. While the fish is baking, prepare your chili-lime sauce. In a small bowl, mix equal parts salsa and Greek yogurt (or drizzle some hot sauce into the Greek yogurt) and a squeeze of lime juice.

4. Make your tacos using a tortilla, the cooked fish, lettuce, chili-lime sauce, and any toppings you enjoy.

Quinoa Sushi *(C, P, F)*

I LIVE for sushi, but find that the rice doesn't do a great job of keeping me satisfied for the long haul. I decided to experiment with quinoa instead, with very satisfying results. The quinoa adds a nutty texture and protein boost to the sushi and is a fun way to change things up.

Makes 4 sushi rolls

> 1 cup quinoa, rinsed
>
> 1 Tb rice vinegar
>
> ½ tsp sugar
>
> ½ tsp salt
>
> 4 sheets nori (you can find these at health food stores and Asian markets)
>
> 4 oz smoked salmon, thinly sliced (*optional*)
>
> 1 avocado, sliced
>
> 1 carrot, julienned
>
> 1 bell pepper, julienned
>
> Tamari and wasabi paste (*optional*) for serving

1. Place the rinsed quinoa into a small saucepan. Add 1½ cups water and salt, bring to a boil, and simmer for about 15 minutes, until quinoa is transparent and has a thin white ring outlining each seed.

2. Stir rice vinegar into the cooked quinoa and allow it to cool to room temperature.

3. Next to your nori sheets, place a small bowl of water. You'll use this to "glue" the nori seam.

4. With seams running horizontal, place one-quarter of the quinoa mixture on the bottom third of the sheet. Add your toppings (veggies, salmon, avocado), and roll away from you, making sure to keep the roll tight.

5. When you get to the end, gently wet your fingertips and smooth each end of the nori sheet to close the seam.

6. Use a very sharp knife to cut your roll into bite-sized pieces.

7. You can make up to four rolls … or if you get tired of rolling (as I often do), make a large sushi salad using the ingredients.

Make Ahead Tip: Make your "sushi rice quinoa" as part of Sunday prep, and chop all of the veggies. When you want to enjoy a sushi roll, grab your nori, add your fillings, and roll up.

Did you know: Nori and other sea vegetables (including arame, wakame, kelp, and dulse) are a fantastic source of iron and iodine. Try sprinkling some on your salad for a salty kick and low-calorie dose of nutrients. They're also anti-inflammatory and high in antioxidants.

Warm Tempeh Salad with Mustard Vinaigrette *(P, F)*

During the winter months, I tend to stray from my salad-loving ways. Warm salads to the rescue! You can still get the comfort of a hot meal, but all of the nutrients a hearty salad can provide. Bonus: some vegetables' nutrients, such as tomatoes', are increased after cooking slightly.

Makes 2 large servings

1 block tempeh, cut into strips

1 red bell pepper, julienned

2 small zucchini, julienned

1 bunch Swiss or rainbow chard (or 2 cups of spinach), ribs removed and leaves torn into bite-sized pieces

Olive oil (or butter)

Pinch of smoked paprika

Sea salt to taste

Pepper to taste

½ cup apple cider vinegar

½ cup canola oil

1 Tb honey

2 cloves garlic, minced

1 Tb Dijon mustard

Splash of hot sauce

¼ tsp salt

⅛ tsp pepper

1. In a large skillet set to medium heat, add some olive oil or butter and the tempeh. Sprinkle the tempeh slices with salt, pepper, and smoked paprika. Cook until browned, at least three minutes on each side.

2. While the tempeh is cooking, prepare your vinaigrette by whisking all ingredients in a small bowl.

3. After the tempeh is browned, push it aside and add a little more oil and the remaining veggies. Cook until the greens have wilted.

4. While the veggies are sautéing—remember to keep them slightly crisp and not mushy—use your wooden spoon or spatula to break the tempeh into smaller pieces.

5. Drizzle the vinaigrette on top (I use about half the mixture and save the rest for salads throughout the week) and lightly toss.

6. Quickly transfer to plates and enjoy!

Sides and dressings

Sides

- Lemon and Garlic Asparagus

- My Favorite Fall Salad with Homemade Vinaigrette

- Quinoa Stuffed Grape Leaves

- Nana's Frijoles

- Polenta Fries

- Smoky and Sweet Potatoes

Lemon and Garlic Asparagus *(N)*

This is our family's go-to green veggie side dish, even though by the time we're ready to eat dinner, the asparagus has already disappeared.

Makes 2–3 servings

> 1 bunch of asparagus, washed and ends trimmed
>
> Olive oil
>
> 2 lemons: one zested and halved (zest reserved), one sliced
>
> 2 to 4 cloves garlic, minced
>
> ¼ cup shredded goat gouda or your favorite hard cheese (*optional*)
>
> Sea salt to taste
>
> Pepper to taste

1. Preheat the oven to 375° F. Spray a roasting dish or glass baking dish with nonstick spray or olive oil.

2. Add your asparagus to the dish and drizzle with olive oil. Season well with salt, pepper, garlic, zest, and shredded cheese. Top with lemon slices and squeeze the juice from the halved lemon on top.

3. Bake for 20 minutes. Enjoy along with your favorite protein and baked sweet potatoes, or chop into a salad or omelet the next day.

Make Ahead Tip: Prep the asparagus with the olive oil, lemon, and seasonings in a container or baggie to store in the fridge. When you get home for dinner, pour into your dish and bake.

My Favorite Fall Salad with Homemade Vinaigrette *(F, C, P)*

This salad combines all the classic flavor of fall, with a bright and slightly sweet vinaigrette.

For vinaigrette (there will be extra to enjoy the rest of the week)

> ½ cup olive oil
>
> ¼ cup balsamic vinegar
>
> 1 Tb honey
>
> 2 cloves garlic, minced

1 tsp Dijon mustard

¼ tsp dried oregano

¼ tsp dried rosemary

¼ tsp sea salt

⅛ tsp pepper

For salad (2 large servings)

2 cups butternut squash or sweet potato (cubed and baked)

4 oz soft goat cheese

2 cups of your favorite salad greens, lightly chopped

¼ cup dried, unsweetened cranberries

¼ cup chopped almonds or walnuts

1. In a large bowl, whisk together the oil, vinegar, honey, garlic, mustard, oregano, rosemary, salt, and pepper for dressing.

2. Add the squash and crumbled goat cheese to the dressing. Top with the salad greens and the dried fruit. Cover in the fridge until you're ready to serve.

3. Add the nuts, toss to combine, and serve.

Tip: Layer the ingredients in Mason jars to store in the fridge (squash first, then cheese, dressing with greens, and dried fruit as the top layer). Keep your nuts in a small snack bag. When you're ready to enjoy, grab the jar, add your nuts, cover, and shake!

Quinoa Stuffed Grape Leaves *(C, P)*

This is a great make-ahead party appetizer or lunch option. Enjoy with grilled protein for a balanced meal.

Makes 2 servings

1 cup cooked quinoa

¼ cup dried apricots, chopped

2 Tb fresh parsley, chopped

1 heaping Tb fresh mint, chopped

1 clove of garlic, finely minced (you can also use ¼ tsp garlic powder if fresh is too intense)

¼ tsp sea salt (more if needed)

⅛ tsp pepper

Pinch of nutmeg

Juice of ½ lemon

Drizzle of olive oil

8 grape leaves (They sell these, usually in a large jar, at most international food markets. I've also seen them at health food stores. If you can't find grape leaves, no worries. These are just as wonderful wrapped in raw Swiss chard with the ribs removed. One chard leaf makes two rolls)

1. Combine the quinoa, apricots, parsley, mint, garlic, salt, pepper, and nutmeg in a large bowl. Squeeze lemon juice on top, drizzle with olive oil, stir well.

2. Place a grape leaf flat on a cutting board and place one-eighth of the quinoa mixture about a half-inch from the bottom of the leaf. Fold the ends in and then roll like a small burrito.

3. Serve in a dish topped with lemon slices.

Nana's Frijoles (C, P)

This is one of our family's favorite recipes. Whenever we would go to nana's house, she'd have fresh beans and homemade tortillas cooking on the stove. While it does take a little longer to cook (it's more of an all-day thing), it's a great component for Sunday meal prep.

1 (16-oz) bag dried pinto beans, rinsed and soaked in water overnight (black beans also work well)

2 heads of garlic, whole, with just the top sliced off

1 Tb oregano

Salt

1. Rinse the soaked beans in a colander. Place in a large pot on the stove, along with the garlic, oregano, and enough water to cover the beans. Salt well.

2. Bring them to a boil and reduce to a simmer. Allow to cook for an hour, until beans are soft. Make sure to keep enough water to cover the beans, so you may have to add more.

3. Taste and add a little more salt as needed. Bring to room temperature and freeze to enjoy later, or enjoy in your make-ahead breakfast burritos, salads, or as a dinner side.

Tip: Soak the beans overnight, and the next morning, rinse well and add to a standard slow cooker with 4 cups water or vegetable broth. Salt well and set the slow cooker on low for six hours.

Polenta Fries *(C)*

This is one of those "recipes that isn't really a recipe," and to be honest, it kind of pushes my buttons when people say, "Try this! It tastes JUST like fries!" Don't lie to me. Your carrots are not fries. But, I have to say ... polenta does kind of taste like fries.

Makes 2–3 servings

    1 (18-oz) tube of polenta

    Dried oregano

    Smoked paprika

    Sea salt to taste

    Pepper to taste

1. Preheat the oven to 375° F and spray a standard cookie sheet with olive oil or nonstick spray.

2. Cut the polenta into French fry shapes and place on the cookie sheet. Season well and bake for 20 minutes until crispy and wonderful.

Smoky and Sweet Potatoes *(C)*

This is an awesome BBQ side dish option. (You know, when the host says, "Maybe bring a side dish?") It's a little different than the usual mashed sweet potatoes and tends to be a huge hit!

Makes 8–10 servings

    8 medium sweet potatoes, baked

    2 Tb butter, melted

    1 to 2 chipotle chilies in adobo, drained and chopped. (Found in the international aisle of most grocery stores. They're in a

small can. Freeze any leftover chilies to add to enchilada sauce or soup. To make this dish less spicy, seed the chilies before adding them.)

¼ cup maple syrup

¼ tsp salt

⅛ tsp pepper

1. Add the sweet potato flesh to the bowl of a large mixer. Mix well until the sweet potatoes are soft and fluffy.

2. Next, add your butter, chilies, maple syrup, salt, and pepper. Taste and adjust seasonings as necessary. If you need to make yourself a small bowl to get the full experience, it's highly recommended.

3. Keep warm in a slow cooker (on low) or store in the fridge to heat and eat throughout the week.

Dressings

- The Best Homemade Balsamic Vinaigrette

- Clean Caesar

- Homemade Lighter Ranch

- Honey, Lemon, and Basil Salad Dressing

The Best Homemade Balsamic Vinaigrette *(F)*

This makes quite a bit of dressing. Make it to enjoy on every salad or as a marinade for protein during the week.

¾ cup olive oil

½ cup balsamic vinegar

2 cloves minced garlic

1 Tb of Dijon mustard

½ tsp Sucanat or brown sugar

½ tsp dried oregano

½ tsp dried thyme

½ tsp salt

⅛ tsp pepper

Whisk all ingredients in a salad dressing shaker or a Mason jar (with the lid tightly attached). Store covered in the fridge.

Clean Caesar *(F)*

Caesar is my favorite salad dressing, but it's usually loaded with unhealthy ingredients. Here is my lighter version, which includes manchego cheese (one of my faves, but you could also use goat gouda or Parmesan), lemon, and anchovies.

Makes 4 servings

4 oz shredded manchego cheese or white, strong cheese of choice

¼ cup olive oil

1 (2-oz) tin of anchovies in olive oil, chopped

Juice of 1 lemon

1 clove garlic

Salt and pepper to taste

1. In a small food processor or blender, combine the cheese, olive oil, anchovies, lemon, and garlic until smooth. Stir in some extra grated cheese for texture, if you like!
2. Pour on your favorite salad greens along with fresh croutons and protein of choice (tempeh, grilled chicken, salmon, and shrimp are all delicious options).

Tip: Store in the fridge for one to two days. For homemade croutons, chop your favorite bread and spray with a little olive oil or coconut oil. Sprinkle with oregano, salt, pepper, and thyme and broil until crispy and golden.

Homemade Lighter Ranch *(N)*

This Ranch dressing is ideal for salads and veggie dipping. I used to be daunted by homemade dressings until I realized how inexpensive and delicious they are. It's worth the extra prep time to know what ingredients are in your salad dressing, plus they taste so much more fresh and vibrant.

Makes 2 large servings

½ cup plain yogurt of choice (I like goat's milk plain yogurt)

2 Tb almond milk

1 Tb apple cider vinegar

1 clove of garlic, finely minced

1 heaping tablespoon fresh parsley, chopped

1 heaping tablespoon fresh dill

½ tsp chives

½ tsp smoked paprika

Splash of hot sauce

Salt and pepper to taste

1. Blend all ingredients in the food processor until you have a smooth consistency. If you need to, add a little more almond milk to get the texture you like.

2. Store, tightly covered in the fridge for three to five days.

Honey, Lemon, Basil Salad Dressing *(F)*

This salad dressing is especially refreshing during the summer months on a salad with greens, chicken, chopped veggies, and a sprinkle of goat or feta cheese.

Makes 6 servings

½ cup olive oil

¼ cup apple cider vinegar

¼ cup fresh basil

2 cloves garlic, minced

1 heaping Tb honey

Sea salt to taste

Pepper to taste

1. Briefly run all ingredients through a blender or mini food chopper.

2. Store in a jar in the fridge to enjoy for your weekly salads, or as a fish or chicken marinade.

Mini meals: snack options that can be enjoyed any time of day

- Chicken Crust Pizza

- BBQ Zucchini Chips

- Chipotle Hummus

- Buffalo Turkey Meatballs

- Savory Butternut Squash Bites

- Popcorn Chicken Bites

- Cookie Dough Bars

- Homemade Grain-Free Granola

- Low-Sugar Granola Bars

- Quinoa Trail Mix Muffins

- Protein Fudge

Chicken Crust Pizza *(P, F)*

I originally made these pizzas to enjoy as part of a recovery meal following a strength training session. The protein in the chicken is an ideal amount, and they can be customized with your favorite pizza toppings. These pizzas also freeze well!

Makes 2 pizzas

1 lb. ground chicken

1 Tb ground flax

1 tsp oregano

½ tsp thyme

½ tsp basil

¼ tsp garlic powder

½ tsp sea salt

¼ tsp pepper

½ cup of your favorite shredded cheese (*optional*)

Your favorite marinara sauce

Pizza toppings

1. Preheat oven to 350° F. Spray a cookie sheet with olive oil or nonstick spray. In a large bowl, combine the chicken, flax, oregano, thyme, basil, garlic, salt, pepper, and cheese if you choose to include it.

2. Separate the meat mixture in half and place the two mounds on the prepared cookie sheet. Using a rolling pin, roll into thin pizza crusts.

3. Bake for 10 minutes. Remove from the oven, add your desired pizza toppings, and bake for an additional 10 minutes.

4. Enjoy with a hearty salad as a protein-packed lunch or dinner!

Make Ahead Tip: Want to make ahead and freeze as part of your Sunday meal prep? Let the pizzas come down to room temperature before freezing in a sealed bag in the freezer. When you're ready to eat, preheat the oven to 400° F and cook for 15 minutes.

BBQ Zucchini Chips *(N)*

These BBQ chips taste exactly like my childhood potato chip fave. It's easy to eat the entire batch in one sitting, and you also get a serving of green veggies. These are fantastic for kids' lunches or to serve along with a lunchtime salad.

Makes ??? servings (depends if you feel like sharing …)

½ tsp smoked paprika

½ tsp chili powder

½ tsp cumin

¼ tsp pepper

¼ tsp salt

½ tsp brown sugar

2 zucchini, cut into long vertical strips using a veggie peeler

1. Whisk together the paprika, chili, cumin, pepper, salt, and brown sugar to create a dry rub.

2. Add the rub mix to the zucchini, and use your hands to make sure each piece is fully coated.

3. If using a dehydrator, place the zucchini strips on Tefflex-lined dehydrator sheets. Dehydrate overnight (flipping at some point) at 118° F. If using a traditional oven, heat the oven to the lowest setting. Cook the zucchini chips on parchment-lined cookie sheets with the door of the oven slightly ajar. This will take a few hours, but it's worth it! The best time to make them is when you know you'll be home for a while.

Make Ahead Tip: I'd give you a tip, but honestly, these bad boys will be gone before you know it. They're a unique snack to pack for kids' lunches, too.

Chipotle Hummus *(C, P)*

This is a smoky twist on a beloved appetizer spread. I especially love it as a salad wrap filling with shredded chicken, sliced carrots, crumbled goat cheese, and spinach. This also makes a wonderful party appetizer with toasted whole-grain pita chips or crudités for dipping.

Makes 6 servings

1 (14-oz) can of garbanzo beans, rinsed and drained

1 or 2 chipotle chilies in adobo sauce (found in the international section of most grocery stores)

Juice of 1 lime

2 cloves garlic

Sea salt to taste

Pepper to taste

Chili powder or smoked paprika to taste (*optional*)

1. Blend the garbanzo beans, chilies, lime, garlic, salt, and pepper in a mini food chopper or blender until smooth.

2. Sprinkle with a little chili powder or smoked paprika, and enjoy with zucchini chips, raw veggies, or your favorite store-bought tortilla chips or whole grain crackers.

Buffalo Turkey Meatballs *(P, F)*

These meatballs make THE BEST meatball sub, and are also delicious on a bed of spiralized zucchini noodles.

Makes 10 meatballs

1 lb. of ground turkey

½ cup almond meal (panko bread crumbs or ground rice crisp cereal works, too!)

1 egg

1 stalk of celery, finely chopped

2 cloves garlic, minced

1 dried oregano

½ tsp smoked paprika

Sea salt to taste

Pepper to taste

4 Tb of your favorite hot sauce (too spicy? use your favorite BBQ sauce instead)

2 Tb grass-fed butter, melted

(you can double the butter and hot sauce amounts to make additional sauce)

1. In a large bowl, combine the turkey, almond meal, egg, oregano, paprika, salt, pepper, garlic, and celery. You may have to use your hands to fully combine. It gets a little messy but it's worth it!

2. Using a melon ball scooper, make 10 meatballs of the same size. Roll with your hands to make sure they don't fall apart.

3. In a large pot on medium-high heat, brown meatballs in olive oil for about 10 minutes or until cooked through.

4. While the meatballs are cooking, combine the hot sauce and butter. Pour on top of the meatballs after checking for doneness. (It's harder to tell if they're cooked through if red sauce is covering them.)

5. Enjoy on top of salad with a sprinkle of goat cheese or blue cheese. You can also pack these in lunches, serve as a party appetizer, or make a buffalo meatball sub. The possibilities are endless!

Tip: You can use the same mixture for Italian meatballs in the slow cooker. Brown the meatballs for five minutes and transfer to the bowl of a slow cooker. Add a jar of your favorite marinara sauce and cook on low for four to five hours. Enjoy on top of salad, with some roasted veggies, or with boiled whole-grain pasta.

Savory Butternut Squash Bites *(C)*

These butternut squash bites are a delicious companion to any of the turkey burgers in the book, or use the leftovers to top a salad.

Makes 4 large servings

24 oz peeled and cubed butternut squash (about 4 cups)

1 tsp chili powder

½ tsp garlic powder

½ tsp cumin

½ tsp paprika

½ tsp Sucanat *(optional)*

¼ tsp sea salt

1. Preheat the oven to 375° F and spray a standard baking sheet with nonstick spray or olive oil.

2. Place your butternut squash on the baking sheet, spray again with olive oil or nonstick spray, and top with your chili, garlic, cumin, paprika, Sucanat, and salt.

3. Bake for 30 minutes, until golden and soft.

Tip: These squash cubes are perfect to make during Sunday prep to add to salads or as a side to an entrée later in the week. I especially love them with sliced avocado and shredded chicken for lunch!

Popcorn Chicken Bites *(P, F)*

I created this version because I wanted a healthy "nugget" option for my daughter when she really started to get into solid food. The recipe is gluten free, surprisingly savory, and dips well in hummus, salsa, ketchup, or your favorite salad dressing.

Makes 2 large servings

  2 medium-size chicken breasts, cut into large bite-sized pieces

  ½ cup almond meal

  ½ cup crushed brown rice cereal

  Garlic powder to taste

  Sea salt to taste

  Pepper to taste

  1 egg

1. Preheat the oven to 375° F. Spray a baking dish with olive oil or nonstick spray. Season the chicken well with salt, pepper, and garlic power.

2. In a separate bowl, add your almond meal and brown rice crumbles, and season with salt, pepper, and garlic powder. Stir to combine.

3. In a small bowl, whisk the egg with 1 Tb of water. Add the chicken cubes to the egg mixture, and toss well to coat. Next, transfer the eggy-chicken to the almond meal and, using a fork, gently toss to coat.

4. Place the chicken bites on your baking dish and bake for 20 minutes until golden and cooked through.

5. Enjoy as a wrap filling or salad topping.

Flavor Variation:

Buffalo kick: Drizzle a mixture of 1 Tb melted butter and 1 Tb hot sauce onto the chicken bites for the last 10 minutes of baking.

Tip: Make a double-batch of these in your Sunday prep to add to meals throughout the week. They also make a protein-packed snack with a healthy dose of fat and fiber from the almond meal.

Cookie Dough Bars *(C, P)*

This is a clean homemade snack bar option and is more cost-effective to make at home than to buy packaged at the store. Feel free to customize by adding dried fruit and/or citrus zest. Kiddos love these bars, too.

Makes 4 bars

> 1 cup raw or roasted almonds
>
> ¼ cup shredded unsweetened coconut
>
> 6 medjool dates, pits removed
>
> ¼ tsp cinnamon
>
> Pinch of sea salt
>
> ¼ cup mini chocolate chips

1. In a small food processor, process the almonds until chopped but not a flour. You still want some texture. Add the coconut, dates, cinnamon, and salt, and pulse until a soft dough forms. Stir in chocolate chips.
2. Press the mixture onto the bottom of a small storage container and place in the fridge to slightly harden, about 1 hour.
3. Cut into 4 bars and store covered in the fridge for up to a week.

Homemade Grain-Free Granola *(F, P, C)*

Despite the arsenal of recipes I like to create, I almost always have eggs for breakfast. My "breakfast" recipes are often enjoyed for lunch when I want a little something sweet, because when it comes to breakfast, I'm all about savory. The only exception: granola. When I get on a granola kick, I'll have a small cup with almond milk, my morning egg or two, and a cup of coffee. This is the staple recipe I make each week, and packaged in a Mason jar and tied with a bow, I also share it with friends.

Makes 6–8 servings

    1 cup almonds

    1 cup walnuts

    ½ cup shredded unsweetened coconut

    ½ cup hemp seeds

    1 tsp vanilla

    ⅓ cup honey

    1 Tb of butter, melted

    Pinch sea salt

    ½ tsp cinnamon

    ½ cup dried fruit

    ¼ to ½ cup mini chocolate chips

1. Preheat the oven to 225° F and line a baking sheet with foil or parchment paper.

2. In a food processor, pulse the almonds and walnuts until chopped. (I like to leave a little bit of texture variation here.) Transfer to a large mixing bowl.

3. Stir in the coconut, hemp seeds, vanilla, honey, butter, and cinnamon. Mix well.

4. Spread the mixture in an even layer on the baking sheet and bake for 45 minutes, stirring once halfway.

5. Let the granola cool completely, and stir in the chocolate chips and dried fruit.

6. Store in the fridge in a sealed container for up to two weeks.

Tip: Can't find hemp seeds? No worries. Chia seeds and flax seeds make great add-in substitutions.

Low-Sugar Granola Bars *(F, P, C)*

As much as we enjoy homemade granola, granola bars are a snack sta-ple in our house. The store-bought varieties can be pricey and/or contain sketchy ingredients, so I prefer to make them here at home. Bonus: I can add as many chocolate chips as I like.

Makes 10 bars

⅓ cup dried apricots

½ cup chopped almonds

½ cup shredded coconut

½ cup raw sunflower seeds

2 Tb chia seeds (can also use ground flax)

½ cup dried cranberries

⅓ cup chocolate chips

½ cup almond meal (can sub more coconut or oat flour)

2 eggs

½ tsp cinnamon

1 tsp vanilla

Pinch of sea salt

1. Preheat the oven to 350° F. Spray an 8-by-8-inch bak-ing pan with nonstick spray or grease with butter or coconut oil.

2. In a small food processor, combine the apricots, coconut, sunflower seeds, chia seeds, cranberries, chocolate chips, and almond meal. Pulse well to chop and combine. Maintain some texture.

3. Transfer the mixture to a large bowl and stir in the eggs, cin-namon, vanilla, and salt. Pour into your baking dish.

4. Bake for 20 minutes, until cooked through. Let cool com-pletely before cutting into bars or squares. Store covered in the fridge for up to one week.

Quinoa Trail Mix Muffins *(C, F, P)*

These trail mix muffins are everything you could wish for: nutty, sweet, filling, and super easy to make. While they're delicious on their own, try one crumbled onto plain yogurt with fresh berries on top.

Makes 7 muffins

> 1 cup quinoa, rinsed
>
> 1 cup almond meal
>
> ½ cup almond milk (or milk of choice)
>
> ¼ cup maple sugar (or brown sugar)
>
> 1 egg
>
> 1 tsp vanilla extract
>
> Pinch of sea salt
>
> ¼ tsp cinnamon
>
> ¼ to ½ cup chocolate chips (I think we all know on which end of the spectrum I fall.)
>
> ¼ cup dried fruit
>
> ¼ cup nuts/seeds of choice (*optional*) (hemp seeds would be amazing)

1. Bring 1¼ cups water to a boil. Reduce heat to low, add quinoa, and cook for 12 minutes. You want the quinoa to be almost cooked, but not super soft and mushy.

2. Preheat the oven to 350° F and spray a 12-cup muffin pan with the nonstick spray or olive oil.

3. Mix all ingredients in a large bowl.

4. Scoop mixture to fill seven muffin tins all the way to the top—these won't be rising.

5. Bake for 25 minutes.

6. The hard part: let them cool completely in the muffin tins before removing. If, like me, patience is not your virtue: scoop one out warm, top with a slice of butter, and enjoy with a fork.

Protein Fudge *(P, F)*

This recipe tastes eerily similar to REAL fudge. Bonus: you can have seconds without the dreaded sugar crash. It's also high in protein, so I love this protein fudge on the go, or as a recovery snack after strength training.

Makes 2 satisfying servings

> 2 scoops (42 g) vanilla or chocolate protein powder of choice (tip: egg-white protein tastes HORRIBLE in this recipe. I'd recommend brown rice or whey protein instead)

> 1 scoop (21 g) coconut flour (ground oat flour would work well, too)

> 2 Tb nut butter of choice (I use sunflower seed butter)

> 1 Tb coconut oil

> *Optional*: sweetener of choice (honey, coconut sugar, and Stevia all work well) to taste

> 1 to 2 Tb cocoa powder (I use 1 Tb, so these have just a touch of chocolate)

> 1 tsp vanilla extract

> Pinch of sea salt

> 1 Tb maple syrup or more (This is going to be dependent on how creamy your nut butter is.)

> 1 Tb chocolate chips

> 1 Tb almond milk

1. Mix the protein powder, coconut flour, nut butter, coconut oil, sweetener, cocoa, vanilla, and salt in a medium bowl, and stir until a dough forms. If the dough is a little too thick, add maple syrup until it reaches the right consistency.

2. Press the mixture into a small storage container and place in the fridge to harden for 15 minutes or so.

3. Melting 2 Tb chocolate chips and 1 Tb almond milk in a glass bowl to make a frosting. You can either use a double

boiler to melt the chocolate chips, or microwave for 20 seconds.

4. Spread the frosting on top of the protein fudge and place in the fridge to harden one more time. Cut into squares and store covered in the fridge.

Flavor variations:

Mint protein fudge: Add ½ to 1 tsp peppermint extract to the fudge mixture.

Berry-lemon protein fudge: Omit the frosting and add 2 Tb fresh or defrosted frozen berries and ½ tsp lemon zest to the fudge mixture.

Chocolate chip protein fudge: A quick option if you'd like to skip the frosting. Just add 1 heaping TB chocolate chips to the fudge mixture.

Peanut butter and jelly protein fudge: Split the fudge in half. Lay the first half flat in your storage container and smear a light layer of jelly on top. Lightly top with the remaining fudge dough.

Juices and drinks

- Tropical Pink Juice

- Carrot, Apple, Beet Detox Juice

- Homemade Almond Milk

- Tropical Refresher

- Chocolate Mint Tea

- Classic Iced Almond Milk Chai

- Iced Coffee

- Apple Pear Ginger Saketini

- Classic Sangria

- Lucky Irish Girl

My Favorite Green Juice *(C)*

I've often heard that green juice can totally replace morning coffee or other types of caffeine (like green tea). For me, this isn't really the case. I need my coffee, but I also appreciate the nutrient-density and energy boost of a fresh juice. I'll often have green juices in the late afternoon as a little pick-me-up. The key to keeping juices from tasting "too green" is a combo of lemon and ginger. This is my go-to green juice recipe! It's bright, energizing, and an easy way to enjoy the benefits of extra produce.

Makes 1 large juice

> 1 English cucumber, washed and roughly chopped
>
> 1 green apple, cut into quarters
>
> ½ lemon with peel intact
>
> Handful of spinach
>
> Pinch of parsley
>
> Stevia to taste

Run all ingredients except the Stevia though a juicer. If needed, add the Stevia to slightly sweeten. This makes a refreshing green lemonade that provides a quick boost of highly bioavailable nutrients and makes skin glow!

Tropical Pink Juice *(C)*

Fresh beet gives this juice a vibrant pink color and also provides a host of health benefits including antioxidants, anti-inflammatory properties, and detoxification. The pineapple makes this a tropical and delicious fresh juice; perfect for juice newbies!

Makes 1 large juice

> 1 cup fresh pineapple
>
> ½ raw red beet
>
> 1 red apple

Run all ingredients through a juicer. Grab a straw and enjoy a tropical getaway with a lovely pink hue.

Carrot, Apple, Beet Detox Juice *(C)*

This is another one of my beloved juice recipes. I would never eat three full, raw carrots, but you can bet that I'll juice them! This juice is slightly sweet, and I like to make it a little spicier with extra ginger. Cheers!

Makes 1 large juice

> 3 carrots
>
> 1 apple
>
> ½ raw beet
>
> Coin of ginger (choose the size depending on how spicy you like it)
>
> ½ English cucumber

Wash all your produce, then run the ingredients through a juicer. Grab a straw and enjoy!

Homemade Almond Milk *(N)*

I'm a huge fan of store-bought almond milk, but I also love the convenience of making my own. It has a fresh and creamy texture and is especially wonderful blended into smoothies or poured on top of granola. Here's the how-to, which is way less intimidating than it may seem.

> 1 cup almonds, soaked at least 1 hour and rinsed
>
> 3 cups water
>
> 1 tsp vanilla
>
> *Optional:* Sweetener of choice (I prefer a little maple syrup. A medjool date works well, too)
>
> ½ tsp cinnamon
>
> Pinch of sea salt

1. Blend all ingredients in a high-speed blender for at least one minute.

2. Attach a fine mesh sieve to the top of a large bowl, and place some cheesecloth across the top.

3. Pour the mixture into the bowl, so that the cheesecloth and sieve double-strain it. You may have to do this in batches, as it drains fairly slowly.

4. Squeeze any excess almond milk out of the cheesecloth.

5. That's it! Store in a sealed container for two days in the fridge.

Flavor Variation:

Chocolate almond milk: Add ¼ to ½ cup cocoa powder.

Tip: Not sure what to do with the leftover almond pulp? Make almond flour! Spread the pulp out in an even layer, either on a cookie sheet (if you'll be using an oven) or a Teflexx sheet for the dehydrator. Cook in the oven on the lowest setting for about an hour, or into the dehydrator overnight. Add the dried flour to the food processor and process until it's a fine mixture. This is the same almond flour I prefer to use in my macaroons!

Tropical Refresher *(C)*

Excellent during the summer months or after a sweaty workout.

Makes 1 large serving

    1½ cups coconut water

    1 cup frozen cubed pineapple

    Juice of half a lime

    1 Tb of fresh mint, chopped

    ½ scoop protein powder *(optional)*

1. Blend all ingredients in a high-speed blender until smooth. If you'd like, add ½ scoop of your favorite vanilla protein powder.

Chocolate Mint Tea *(N)*

This is a recipe that isn't really a recipe per se, but rather a combo of two of my favorite things.

Makes 1 serving

    1 cup chocolate milk

    1 bag mint tea

Heat a mug of your favorite chocolate milk (I enjoy the chocolate almond milk) in the microwave for one to two minutes. Add a mint tea bag and allow to steep for at least five minutes. Heat the milk again if you need to, then add a little Stevia or sweetener of choice.

Classic Iced Almond Milk Chai *(N)*

A sweet and spiced drink, and it's even better made the night before!

Makes 4 large servings

4 cups water

¼ cup of fresh ginger, sliced

10 cardamom pods, gently crushed

6 whole black peppercorns

6 whole cloves

4 cinnamon sticks

3 star anise

1 vanilla bean, sliced down the middle

Large pinch of nutmeg

1 Tb brown sugar

4 black tea bags

4 cups almond milk or cold milk of choice

Pinch ground cinnamon

Sweetener to taste (*optional*)

1. In a large saucepan, bring the water to a boil. Next, add all of your spices, tea, and sugar, turn the heat off, and allow to come to room temperature (about four hours).

2. Strain the mixture into a large pitcher, and then stir in your milk. Store covered in the fridge for up to five days.

3. When you're ready to enjoy, pour into a glass with some ice (optional), a sprinkle of ground cinnamon, and some sweetener if you like.

Iced Coffee *(N)*

This iced coffee lasts for about a week when covered in the fridge, and it is much more cost-effective than buying the canned cuppa joe. Bonus: it's delicious in a smoothie or as your liquid when cooking oatmeal.

Makes 10 servings

> 1 (8.8-oz) container of ground espresso (I love the Illy brand)
>
> 10 cups cold water
>
> Cheesecloth and fine mesh sieve

1. Add the coffee grounds to the water in a large bowl, and let soak, covered, overnight.
2. The next morning, strain the mixture using cheesecloth placed over a fine mesh sieve.
3. Add the mixture back to a large pitcher or covered container and store in the fridge.
4. When you're ready to enjoy, pour a glass and mix with almond milk, your favorite sweetener, and a sprinkle of cinnamon. Cheers!

Cocktails

If you choose to imbibe, it can be a part of a healthy lifestyle. I have a small glass of red wine almost every night with dinner. The key is to choose beverages that are naturally low in sugar or that can boost a little antioxidant power. Here are a couple of my favorite cocktail recipes that are perfect for parties with friends or your next girls' night.

Apple Pear Ginger Saketini *(T)*

This fresh cocktail pairs nicely with Asian dishes (such as my slow cooker cashew chicken or quinoa sushi) and is perfect for fall dinner parties.

Makes 1 serving

> ½ cup ice
>
> 1 cup of pear, apple, ginger juice (I use 1 large apple, 1 large pear, and a large coin of ginger for 8 oz). If you don't have a

juicer, you can use store-bought juice. Just mix apple, pear, and add a coin of ginger to infuse the flavor.

2 shots (3 oz) sake of choice

⅓ cup lemon sparkling water

1. Shake ice, juices, and sake in a cocktail shaker. Pour into a glass and top with sparkling water.

Classic Sangria *(T)*

This is one of my standard summer BBQ (OK, or any occasion) *cocktail recipes. It's easily made the day before the party, and is frequently requested for friend and family get-togethers.*

Makes 6 servings

  2 green apples, thinly sliced

  2 oranges: one sliced, one juiced

  1 sliced lemon

  2 Tb sugar

  ½ cup orange juice

  ½ cup brandy

  ½ cup triple sec

  2 bottles of inexpensive red wine. Inexpensive wine is the key here! No reason to use hoity-toity wine. The inexpensive stuff tastes even better in sangria.

1. In a large pitcher, add the apple slices, oranges, lemon, juice, brandy, sugar, and triple sec. Stir to combine.

2. Pour in the red wine and stir well.

3. Allow to sit in the fridge overnight so the flavors can party.

4. When you're ready to enjoy, serve over ice and garnish with a long strand of orange zest or a lemon wedge.

Lucky Irish Girl *(T)*

This is my most decadent cocktail recipe, but it's fantastic for a treat or special occasion. (We also sometimes have it colored green for St. Patrick's Day.) This is a recipe that was handed down from my husband's father, and while he makes it the best (with heavy cream, of course), this is my lighter version. Also, if you're sharing it with dudes, feel free to change the name.

Makes 1 serving

> 1 oz Irish cream liqueur, such as Baileys
>
> ½ oz coffee liqueur, such as Kahlua
>
> ½ oz hazelnut liqueur, such as Frangelico
>
> 2 oz milk of choice (I use almond or coconut)

1. Mix all ingredients in a cocktail shaker with a little ice.
2. Shake it! Serve it.

Chapter 9

Sweet Treats

One of my favorite things to do is health-ify my favorite treats. I like to enjoy splurge treats occasionally, but it's fun to experiment with whole ingredients as I re-create the classic faves. When the sweet tooth comes knocking, here are some of my all-time favorite treat recipes. They use whole ingredients, unrefined sugars, and many are gluten and/or dairy free. While they're technically healthier options, you'd never guess. Put them on your next party dessert tray and watch them disappear …

- Almond Butter Chocolate Chip Cookies
- Black Forest Cupcakes
- Cinnamon Apple Tartlets
- Blueberry Muffin Bake
- Quinoa Cookies
- Brown Rice Crunch Squares
- Mixed Berry Crumble
- Flourless Dark Chocolate Cookies
- Pumpkin Chocolate Chip Bread
- Sweet Potato Gluten-Free Brownies
- Classic Vegan Macaroons

Almond Butter Chocolate Chip Cookies *(T)*

This is one of my most popular blog recipes. It's whole grain, vegan, and you would never know!

Makes 12 cookies

- 2 cups spelt flour, or your favorite gluten-free mix
- 2 tsp baking powder
- 1½ tsp cinnamon
- ½ tsp baking soda
- ½ tsp sea salt
- ½ cup chocolate chips
- ¾ cup pure maple syrup
- ½ cup raw almond butter (crunchy or creamy. I use TJs creamy)
- ¼ cup canola oil
- 1½ Tb vanilla extract
- 1 tsp molasses

1. Preheat the oven to 350° F and line a standard cookie sheet with parchment paper.
2. Combine the flour, baking powder, cinnamon, baking soda, and salt until thoroughly mixed, and then add your chocolate chips. Stir to combine.
3. Combine the maple syrup, almond butter, canola oil, vanilla, and molasses in a separate bowl and add to the dry ingredients. Form ball-shaped pieces of dough into slightly flattened cookies on the baking sheet. The mix will be sticky, so do what you can.
4. Bake for 11 minutes, remove from oven and allow the cookies to remain on the baking sheet for one minute longer, then transfer to wire racks to cool.

Flavor Variation: These pizza cookies are the best way to enjoy the almond butter chocolate chip cookies.

Makes 6 servings

　　1 batch of almond butter chocolate chip cookie dough (page 266)

　　Your favorite vanilla ice cream (I especially love Laloo's goat's milk ice cream and So Delicious's dairy-free frozen coconut milk)

　　Chocolate chips for serving

1. Separate the dough into six equal servings (or four … or two …) and put them into ramekins or small cast iron skillets. Lightly spray with olive oil or nonstick cooking spray. You can also put all the dough in one cast iron skillet and serve from there. As you can tell, it's totally flexible.

2. Here's the idea: you underbake the cookie (it's OK because it's vegan) and then top with ice cream and serve. For the almond butter cookie recipe, split into six servings, Cook about 15 minutes at 350° F. Top with ice cream, chocolate chips, and serve.

Girls' Night Tip: This is the *best* with cocktails (check out the cocktail section for ideas). Homemade pizza, salad, and a pizza cookie: Perfection!

Black Forest Cupcakes *(T)*

This grain-free cupcake recipe is a decadent dessert, especially when topped with some coconut milk ice cream.

Makes 6–8 cupcakes

　　¾ cup shredded coconut, ground into flour (reduces to about ¼ cup)

　　⅔ cup almond meal

　　¼ cup cocoa powder

　　1 tsp cinnamon

　　½ tsp baking soda

　　Pinch of sea salt

　　2 eggs

¼ cup + 2 Tb honey

½ cup dried Bing cherries

¼ cup mini chocolate chips

1. Preheat your oven to 325° F and prepare a 12-cup muffin tin with cupcake liners.

2. In a mixing bowl, combine the coconut, almond meal, cinnamon, sea salt, cocoa powder, and baking soda. Whisk to combine.

3. Next, add the eggs and honey and mix well. Stir in the cherries and chocolate chips.

4. Scoop batter into muffin cups and bake for 30 minutes, until fluffy and set.

Tip: These are especially delicious crumbled into vanilla yogurt with fresh berries and a sprinkle of hemp seeds.

Cinnamon Apple Tartlets *(T)*

This recipe is a beautiful make-ahead dessert option for dinner parties. Cover, put in the fridge overnight, and the next evening all you have to do is bake and top with ice cream. These tartlets are grain free, refined-sugar free, and totally delicious.

Makes 4 large servings

6 apples, peeled and sliced (this is the most annoying part)

Juice of ½ lemon

½ tsp cinnamon

⅛ tsp nutmeg

⅛ tsp cloves

Pinch of sea salt

1½ cups almond meal (you can also grind almonds in a high-powered blender or food processor to make your own)

2 medjool dates, pitted

¼ cup pure maple syrup

½ tsp vanilla

2 Tb melted butter or coconut oil

1. Preheat the oven to 350° F. Lightly butter a pie dish or spray with nonstick spray.

2. In a medium bowl, combine the apples with spices, lemon juice, and a pinch of sea salt.

3. In a food processor, combine the almond meal, dates, maple syrup, and vanilla until a soft dough forms.

4. Gently press the dough onto the bottom of the pie dish and top with the sliced apples. Drizzle with coconut oil or butter.

5. Bake for 25 minutes until golden brown, bubbly, and delicious. For a more intense foodgasm experience, serve with coconut milk vanilla ice cream.

Blueberry Muffin Bake *(T)*

This grain-free and flour-free recipe is a perfect breakfast treat; light, creamy, and a bright flavor from fresh lemon zest.

Makes 4 large servings

½ cup creamy almond butter

2 eggs

1 tsp coconut sugar

1 tsp lemon zest

1 tsp vanilla extract

¾ tsp cinnamon

⅛ tsp nutmeg

¼ tsp baking soda

Pinch of sea salt

1 cup fresh blueberries (you can also use thawed frozen blueberries)

1. Preheat the oven to 350° F and spray a 9-inch loaf pan with nonstick spray.

2. In a large bowl, use a fork to whisk the almond butter until fluffy and creamy. Whisk in the eggs.

3. Stir in the coconut sugar, lemon zest, vanilla extract, cinnamon, baking soda, and salt, and mix to combine. Carefully fold in blueberries.

4. Pour the mixture into your prepared loaf pan.

5. Bake for 20 to 25 minutes and allow to cool before storing, covered in the refrigerator.

Tip: Enjoy this warm with a smear of organic butter, along with an egg in the morning. It's a lovely breakfast option or sweet afternoon treat.

Quinoa Cookies *(T)*

These quinoa cookies are perfect to have on hand when the sweet tooth strikes. They have a unique texture from the quinoa grains, plus a dose of protein and healthy fats. They're a satisfying sweet treat, and are especially lovely crumbled onto your favorite coconut milk ice cream.

Makes 12 small cookies

2 cups cooked quinoa

½ cup almond butter

⅓ cup maple syrup

½ cup mini chocolate chips

¼ cup cocoa powder

¼ cup dried fruit (*optional*)

¼ cup nuts (*optional*)

1 tsp vanilla

Pinch of sea salt

1. In a large bowl, combine the ingredients until well mixed.

2. Using a melon ball scoop, scoop the mixture and flatten with your hands to create cookie shapes. Place the cookies on parchment paper in a freezer storage container or on a covered plate.

3. Put the cookies in the freezer to harden for at least 30 minutes. Store covered in the fridge.

Brown Rice Crunch Squares *(T)*

Word to the wise: good luck getting these into the fridge. The batter is very delicious.

Makes 10

> 4 cups crisp brown rice cereal
>
> ¾ cup honey
>
> ¾ cup creamy almond butter or peanut butter
>
> 2 Tb butter
>
> 1 tsp vanilla
>
> 1 tsp cinnamon
>
> Pinch of sea salt

1. Spray a 9 × 13-inch baking dish with nonstick spray.
2. Place the cereal into a large mixing bowl.
3. In a medium-small saucepan, heat the butter on medium low until melted, and stir in the nut butter, honey, cinnamon, vanilla, and sea salt. Stir until fully combined and creamy.
4. Pour the liquid mixture over the cereal and stir well to fully coat.
5. Press the mixture into the baking dish, and use the back of a spoon to flatten. Allow to harden covered in the fridge (about 30 minutes) before cutting into squares.

Mixed Berry Crumble *(T)*

This is one of my husband's frequent dessert requests, and we especially love it during the summer using fresh berries from the farmers' market. Make extra to store in the fridge and you can quickly reheat and top with ice cream for a sweet treat.

Makes 4 servings

> ½ cup old-fashioned oats (or gluten-free oats)
>
> ½ cup almond meal
>
> 3 Tb brown sugar or Sucanat

2 Tb butter, cold and chopped into small pieces

½ tsp cinnamon

½ tsp vanilla

Pinch of sea salt

1½ cups fresh or frozen berries

1 tsp sugar or sugar substitute

½ tsp lemon zest

Juice of half a lemon

1. Preheat the oven to 350° F and spray two Mason jars or a 9-inch loaf pan with nonstick spray. (I use the pint-sized jars, but if you use larger or smaller, adjust the recipe accordingly. This is one of those beautiful things where you don't have to be super precise; you can easily use ratios you prefer.)

2. In a large bowl, combine the oats, almond meal, brown sugar, cinnamon, vanilla, and sea salt. Using a fork, smash in the butter until it is crumbled into the mixture. Set aside.

3. In another bowl, combine the berries, sugar, lemon juice, and zest.

4. Layer the berry mixture with the crumble mixture in the prepared jars or loaf pan. Bake for 30 minutes or until gloriously browned and bubbly.

Flourless Dark Chocolate Cookies *(T)*

Chocoholics, rejoice!

Makes 10–12 small cookies

2 cups Sucanat or coconut sugar

½ cup cocoa powder

¼ tsp cinnamon

¼ tsp espresso powder

2 egg whites

1 tsp vanilla extract

Pinch of sea salt

½ cup chocolate chips

1. Preheat the oven to 350° F and line two cookie sheets with silpat or parchment paper.

2. Briefly blend the Sucanat or coconut sugar in a high-speed blender to create a softer texture, similar to powdered sugar. A few good pulses should do the trick.

3. Add the "powdered sugar" to a large bowl and stir in the remaining ingredients. It will look like thin cake batter, but trust that it will bake beautifully.

4. Using a melon ball scooper, scoop tablespoon-sized amounts onto the cookie sheet. Leave 2 inches between each one because they'll spread out as they bake.

5. Bake for 13 to 15 minutes until set and slightly cracked. Let cool completely (this is key!) before using a spatula to remove the cookies from the cookie sheet.

Pumpkin Chocolate Chip Bread *(T)*

A festive fall loaf. Perfect to wrap up with a bow and take to work ... if you feel like sharing.

Makes 1 loaf

1½ cups brown rice flour

½ cup almond meal (or oat flour)

2 tsp baking powder

2 tsp cinnamon

½ tsp nutmeg

¼ tsp sea salt

1 (3.5-oz) bar dark chocolate (I use the kind with cacao nibs), chopped (Your call on this one. You can use less, but I say go big or go home.)

½ can (7.5-oz, about ½ cup) pumpkin puree

½ to ¾ cup Sucanat (or brown sugar) depending on how sweet you want it

½ cup milk of choice

2 flax eggs (2 Tb ground flax soaked with 4 Tb water)

1 tsp vanilla

1 tsp molasses

1. Preheat the oven to 350° F and grease a 9-inch loaf pan with butter or nonstick spray.
2. In a large bowl, combine the flour, baking powder, sea salt, cinnamon, and nutmeg and whisk to "sift." Add the chopped chocolate and stir.
3. Next, add in the pumpkin puree, sugar, milk, vanilla, molasses, and flax eggs and mix to fully incorporate all the goods.
4. Bake in a loaf pan for 30 minutes, then remove, cover with foil, and bake an additional 15 minutes. A toothpick inserted in the middle should come out clean. Let cool, then slice and serve.

Sweet Potato Gluten-Free Brownies *(T)*

Get your sweet treat and serving of vegetables in one fix. You'd never guess that sweet potatoes give these brownies a sweet flavor and luscious texture.

Makes 6 servings

1 (3.5-oz) bar dark chocolate

1½ Tb coconut oil

¼ cup cocoa powder

1 Tb vanilla

½ tsp cinnamon

¼ tsp espresso powder (can be omitted, but I think it gives brownies a richer taste)

Flesh of two medium-small sweet potatoes (a little under 2 cups); give them a whirl through the food processor for a smoother texture

1 egg

2 Tb ground flax

¼ cup pure maple syrup

¼ cup gluten-free flour blend (or flour of choice)

½ tsp baking powder

Hefty pinch of sea salt

1. Preheat oven to 325° F and grease a 9-inch pie dish with olive oil.

2. Melt the chocolate with the coconut in a double-boiler or in the microwave (check and stir after 20-second intervals).

3. Add in the cocoa powder and stir until there are no lumps or chunks of powdery magma.

4. Next, stir in the vanilla, cinnamon, espresso powder, and mix well, then add the sweet potatoes, egg, flax, and maple syrup.

5. Sift the flour, baking powder, and salt into the wet ingredients and stir to combine.

6. Pour mixture into the pie dish (This is where I save a little in the bowl to enjoy. Salmonella schmalmonella.) and bake for about 25 minutes until a toothpick inserted in the center comes out clean.

Classic Vegan Macaroons

This is my all-time signature dessert, and one that I've been making on the blog for years. It may also be the reason that many of you purchased this book, because I'm finally spilling the beans on the recipe. These vegan macaroons are crunchy on the outside and soft on the inside, and they can be made in a variety of flavors.

Makes 12–15 macaroons

2½ cups shredded, unsweetened coconut

1 cup almond meal (or make your own almond flour by dehydrating almond pulp leftover from homemade almond milk)

1 cup maple syrup

⅓ cup coconut oil

1 Tb honey (or replace with maple syrup)

¼ tsp cinnamon

Large pinch of sea salt

1. If you have a dehydrator, grab two dehydrator sheets and set aside. If you're using the oven, preheat to 200° F, or your oven's lowest setting, and line a standard cookie sheet with parchment paper.

2. Combine all ingredients in a standard mixer, and mix well until a soft dough forms. A hand-mixer or bowl and spoon work well, too; just use lots of elbow grease and make sure everything is fully combined.

3. Using a melon ball scooper, scoop macaroon "balls" onto either your dehydrator sheets or cookie sheet.

4. If dehydrating, set the temperature to 118° F and allow to dehydrate for two days. This is a tragedy, but you may have to test a few along the way for quality control and to determine how crisp you'd like the outside. If cooking in the oven, place the cookie sheet on the middle rack and leave the door slightly ajar. (Of course, make these when you'll be home for a few hours.) Cook until set completely.

Flavor Variations:

Chocolate: Add ⅓ cup cocoa powder or ½ cup raw cacao powder.

Mocha: Add ⅓ cup cocoa powder or ½ cup raw cacao powder and 1 tsp espresso powder.

Chocolate peanut butter: Add ⅓ cup cocoa powder or ½ cup raw cacao powder. Next, stir in ½ cup peanut butter into the dough until the mixture is gently swirled.

Meyer lemon: Add 1 tsp fresh Meyer lemon zest and the juice of the lemon to the dough.

Blueberry lavender: Add ½ cup fresh or dried blueberries and 1 tsp dried lavender.

Super roon: Add ½ cup dried goji berries, ¼ cup cacao nibs, and 1 heaping Tb maca powder.

Red velvet: Add ⅓ cup cocoa powder and ¼ cup fresh beet juice (for red color).

Chapter 10

Prep for Success

One of the most efficient strategies for success is to plan ahead for the week. The weeks that I haven't planned or made some meals or snacks are the ones where I find myself diving into something unhealthy because I'm hungry and it's the most convenient option. The key is to make healthy choices as convenient as possible. Not only will you feel a lot better from eating clean foods, but you'll also find yourself looking forward to enjoying the treats you've made.

So how in the world do I have time to prepare meals in advance? I don't spend a lot of time doing it. The more you practice, the easier the process becomes, and you quickly realize how much you can accomplish! I'll give myself one hour on Sunday nights to prep as many options as possible for the week. I have a checklist of the things I'd like to make, the ingredients and recipes on hand and ready to go, and I take a look at the clock and go for it. When the hour is over, I stop working. Usually, I'll make just as much as I'd anticipated, and enough to get us through most of our meals and snacks.

Prep ahead strategies

Quinoa

Quinoa is a fantastic prepared grain option. I'll cook mine in the rice cooker (on the "brown rice" setting) and make a large enough batch to enjoy for the week.

Make sure to rinse the quinoa before preparing it, as it's coated with a chemical that prevents birds from feasting on the lovely grain, and be sure it's cooked completely before storing. You can tell the quinoa is finished when it's soft, translucent, and has a small white line running through each grain.

Some ways to use your cooked quinoa

- **As a salad topping.** Quinoa, balsamic dressing, salad greens, goat cheese, and chicken (or tempeh) make a perfect lunch salad.

- **Try healthy "fried" quinoa.** In a large pan, sauté some veggies in a little grass-fed butter, ghee, or coconut oil, and then add an egg. Scramble the egg with the veggies, and when it's fully cooked add your serving of quinoa. Pour in a drizzle of tamari, some garlic powder, and *boom*: healthy takeout at home.

- **Fluff up some quinoa with your favorite salad dressing, dried fruit, and nuts.** I especially love quinoa, chopped almonds, and dried cranberries; a delightful sweet and savory pairing.

- **Use it in quinoa pancakes or muffins.** Check out the recipe section for a couple of quinoa baked goodies. You can store the muffins to reheat during the week with breakfast or as a snack option.

- **Breakfast quinoa!** Heat some up in the morning with almond milk, then add chopped banana or berries, cinnamon, Stevia or coconut sugar, and a sprinkle of nuts. It's a filling and delicious breakfast porridge.

Veggie prep

For me, the hardest part about *using* the produce I buy is the act of preparing it. I'll think about the zucchini in the produce drawer, and the labor involved to chop it, and guess what? I take the same zucchini out of the produce drawer two weeks later to find it bruised, wrinkled, and sad looking. This is why I find it so helpful to chop as much as I can in advance. If I know I'm going to be peeling and chopping a few ingredients, it's easier to hype myself up about the task at hand. I play some music, wash and chop as many veggies as possible, and store them in the fridge. This way, I'm that much closer to salad victory when lunch time rolls around.

Another way to enjoy veggies is to roast a large batch to enjoy for the week. Chop your favorite mix of vegetables. Anything goes!

I especially love zucchini, squash, asparagus, tomatoes, and sweet potato. Drizzle with ghee, coconut oil, or a little melted grass-fed butter, and season with salt, pepper, garlic powder, rosemary, and thyme. Bake on a cookie sheet for about 40 minutes, until they reach your desired texture. This is the pizazz at the end: when they're finished, add fresh lemon zest and the juice of an entire lemon. Toss to coat and if you like, add fresh chopped basil. Veggie perfection! (I find that they're best consumed within five days before soggy city sets in).

Some ways to use your raw prepared veggies

- **In stir fries**. Sauté on the stove top with your favorite lean protein and smart fat. Try a mix of veggies (such as bell pepper, onion, or broccoli) with some salmon or tempeh and a splash of tamari.

- **Fast salads!** Add your salad ingredients to a glass jar and store in the fridge. I like to layer the toppings according to moisture status—chopped veggies, grains, and protein on the bottom, greens on the top—and when you're ready to eat, add your dressing, put the lid back on, and shake! Perfect for salads-on-the-go.

Some ways to use your roasted veggies

- **For quiches.** Add your cooked veggies to the bottom of a greased baking dish. Top with your favorite cheese (I'm on a huge manchego kick!), your egg mixture (six eggs with 1 Tb of milk, salt, and pepper work nicely), and a sprinkle of smoked paprika. Bake for about 30 minutes at 325° F (until golden brown and set) and serve with a salad.

- **Add to eggs and omelets.** Cook your eggs in a pan, then add your veggies. Scramble it up and top with avocado slices or add roasted veggies to your omelet, wrap in a brown rice tortilla, and drizzle with hot sauce.

- **Stir fry them up!** Chop and cook your favorite protein in a large skillet. When it's *thisclose* to being done, toss in your refrigerated cooked vegetables. Splash with a little tamari, garlic, and sriracha (if you like it spicy!) and dinner is served.

- **Add to a wrap.** Wrap in a whole-grain tortilla with hummus and a little chicken or tempeh. Drizzle with balsamic vinegar.

Fruit Prep

The beauty about fruit prep is that there's not much to do in advance. I like to wash and chop berries to store in a clear container. Apples and pears can be stored with a squeeze of lemon juice to prevent browning, and most stone fruits (such as peaches, apricots, and plums) keep well chopped in the fridge. Fruit is nature's candy! Try to expand your fruit horizons by trying something new each week.

How to use your washed, chopped fruit

- **Build a parfait:** Layer fruit in a glass with Greek yogurt and granola (check out the recipe on pages 251–252). Top with a sprinkle of sunflower or hemp seeds.

- **Add to yogurt, smoothies, or morning oats.**

- **Toss into a salad.**

- **Fresh trail mix:** Add a serving of almonds, a sprinkle of dried coconut, and enjoy.

Sweet potatoes

OK, technically sweet potatoes are a vegetable, but I use them so much they need their own category! Sweet potatoes provide a filling combination of smart carbs and fiber. They are high in beta-carotene and provide a host of nutritional benefits. They're also easy to prep ahead and enjoy the rest of the week. I'll bake an entire bag of sweet potatoes, knowing that my daughter and I will finish them before the week is up. They're lovely with lunches (chicken, black bean, and sweet potato is a match made in heaven), breakfasts (with eggs!), or especially amazing in sweet potato brownies (see the recipe on page 274).

During Sunday prep, wash as many sweet potatoes as you'd like to consume for the next five days. Poke the sweet potatoes with a fork, and place on a baking dish in the oven at 375° F. About an hour later, they should be pleasantly soft. Let cool to room temperature before storing covered in the fridge. If you're going to use them for mashed sweet potatoes, peel them while they're still warm; it's easier to get the skin off that way.

How to use your prepped sweet potatoes

- **In a smoothie.** It seems like a strange idea, but they add a sweet flavor and smooth texture to pumpkin pie-esque smoothies. In your blender, combine 1½ cups milk of choice, ½ banana, ½ medium sweet potato, 1 scoop of protein powder, ¼ tsp cinnamon, a pinch of nutmeg, and a pitted medjool date. Blend and enjoy!

- **Stuffed sweet potatoes.** The options are endless! I enjoy a Southwestern twist with grilled chicken, black beans, guacamole, and salsa. Some other fave combos include the following:

  - Goat cheese and chives: Crumble one serving of goat cheese, sprinkle with salt and some fresh chopped chives.

  - Tropical style: With chopped pineapple, cucumber, bell pepper, cilantro, and a spicy almond butter dressing.

  - With roasted veggies and ginger miso dressing (see page 220)

  - Dessert style with a sprinkle of cinnamon, coconut sugar, and a drizzle of almond butter

- **In baked goodies.** The brownies on page 274 are one of my all-time fave sweet potato uses.

- **For breakfast.** Top with an egg and some salad and it's a filling, sweet and savory start to the day.

- **Chopped and add to salads for lunch.** Try baked sweet potato with goat cheese, salad greens, balsamic dressing, and fresh sliced basil.

- **Sweet potato nachos!** I'll slice baked sweet potatoes up like chips, or bake them (20 minutes at 350° F, thinly sliced) and top with black beans, salsa, goat cheese, and/or sliced avocado.

- **As a quick dinner component.** If I have chopped veggies and baked sweet potatoes already on hand, I can quickly scramble an egg or prep some protein for a well-rounded meal.

Frozen faves

Some of our most-frequent meals have at one point lived in the freezer, and you'd never know the difference. It's so much easier to make a large batch of something and freeze the rest to enjoy later. Don't tell anyone, mmm k? It can be our little secret.

Some tips for freezer storage

- **Invest in good containers.** Plastic doesn't seem to work very well—I prefer glass containers because they're oven safe—but plastic baggies are ideal for liquids and soups. Bonus: you can wash the plastic baggies in the dishwasher and reuse them.

- **Make sure to allow your food to come to room temperature before freezing.** This helps to prevent freezer burn and bacteria build-up.

- **Avoid room for air between the food and the container.** Pick a container that's the approximate size of what you'd like to store. This will help to minimize freezer burn, and you won't be using more valuable freezer space than necessary.

- **Don't freeze items that were once frozen, thawed, and previously used.** One time in the freezer and that's it.

Some of my favorite freezer staples

- **Perfect protein pancakes.** In the morning, put them in the toaster and pop! Breakfast is done.

- **Quiches.** They reheat nicely, and are a great way to use leftover vegetables from dinner.

- **Chilis and soups.** Pour leftover soup or chili into a large bag—try folding the sides down before pouring, as it keeps the "zipper" part from getting covered in soup—flatten and seal. Store these flat in the freezer and they'll take up less room.

- **Breakfast burritos.** These are amazing for breakfast-in-a-pinch. Make your favorite egg burritos (Southwestern-style with black beans, salsa, and avocado; classic with goat cheese and sweet potato; veggie with mixed vegetables and tempeh bacon), wrap individually in foil, and place in a large plastic bag. When you want to enjoy one, remove from the foil, place on a glass plate, and microwave for two to three minutes.

- **Chicken crust or zucchini pizzas** (see pages 245 and 219). These keep well in the freezer and are wonderful with a large salad for lunch or dinner.

- **Smoothie packs.** You can get as creative as you'd like with this one! Since smoothies don't freeze particularly well—they defrost like an awkward sludge—I prefer to freeze the ingredients for each smoothie in a small baggie. This way, in the morning, all I have to do is add the liquid ingredients, protein powder if I'm feelin' it, and blend it up. Pour into a glass, grab a straw, and bottoms up, buttercup! See pages 191 to 192 for lots of flavor suggestions.

Protein punches

Protein is a critical component of meal prep success. Ideally, you want to choose a versatile protein option that you enjoy, whether you're of the carnivore or plant-based mentality.

Some protein options
- **Chicken or turkey:** Breasts or drumsticks are both versatile choices to have in the fridge. It's common to enjoy prepared meat for up to one week, but I try to consume the premade protein within three to five days max. I'll ask the husband to grill some chicken breasts that I can chop and add to salads, omelets, wraps, and stir fries during the week.

Quick and easy protein seasonings

Mexican flair: Oregano, cumin, chili powder, lime juice, and lime zest.

Tropical: Orange juice and zest, chopped pineapple, veggies, and chili powder.

Savory: Thyme, rosemary, garlic, basil, and oregano.

Spiced: Cumin, coriander, cinnamon, garam masala, and turmeric, which has anti-inflammatory properties.

Asian inspired: Drizzle a little tamari or Nama Shoyu, garlic powder, cayenne, fresh minced ginger, and sesame oil.

Maple-Dijon: Combine 2 Tb maple syrup with 1 tsp Dijon. Sprinkle in salt and pepper, and add a squeeze of orange juice.

Blackened: Equal parts (try ½ tsp of each) cumin, smoked paprika, chili powder, oregano, garlic powder, and coconut sugar (brown sugar is great, too). Mix well, then add a little salt and pepper.

- **Chicken salad:** This is a wonderful wrap/sandwich filler or salad topper. For this one, I'll chop two chicken breasts. In a small bowl, I'll combine ½ mashed avocado, ½ cup plain goat's milk Greek yogurt, ½ tsp yellow curry powder, salt, pepper, ¼ cup chopped walnuts, some chopped scallions, and ½ cup halved red grapes. Add this to the chopped chicken and it's a much lighter version of the classic fave. The avocado adds a beautiful creamy texture, too.

- **Tempeh bacon:** I'm not a huge fan or advocate of soy products, but tempeh is fermented and found to be less estrogenic than the nonfermented varieties. If you enjoy soy products in your diet, be sure to purchase organic non-GM tempeh, as soy is one of the most common genetically modified foods. (Remember, aim for whole foods, not science experiments.) For your tempeh bacon, you'll slice the tempeh up into thin "bacon" strips and place in a bowl. Top the strips with ¼ cup tamari, 1 Tb olive oil, ½ tsp each of garlic powder, cumin, smoked paprika, brown sugar, salt, and ¼ tsp pepper. Heat a large skillet to medium heat, add some ghee or coconut oil, and fry until crispy. Tempeh bacon makes eggs sing with happiness and is also the star of homemade vegan BLT sandwiches.

- **Steamed eggs:** Hard-boiling eggs used to freak me out. This was because I always managed to over- or undercook them and it left our house smelling like death for the rest of the day. Remedy: The steamer. Add some water to a large pot and bring it up to boil, place the steamer basket and your eggs inside. Cover and steam for 15 minutes—perfect eggs every time, and no need to go fishing through boiling hot water for the eggs. Enjoy them for breakfast, with a snack, or in some homemade egg salad. Or, even better: use them with your tempeh bacon to make a killer Cobb salad.

Food gadgets

All you need to make a delicious healthy meal is some fresh ingredients, maybe a bowl, and a little bit of gusto. The tools don't make the cook! But, there are a few gadgets that can make prep a little bit easier. Here are some of my standard kitchen tools, which vary in expense. You can find most of these gadgets for $20 to $40, and they can be helpful investments in your family kitchen.

- **Mini food chopper.** You can get all fancy pants with a large food chopper, but I like the smaller versions for storage purposes. Anything with an "S" blade will do for pureeing hummus, pâtés, chopping veggies, and blending dressings.

- **Blender.** A high-speed blender can be an invaluable food gadget, especially if you're a smoothie fan. High-speed blenders are on the spendy side, but are great investments if you use them often. Check out your local wholesale warehouse or Black Friday deals if you're planning on checking one out! You can make almost anything in a high-speed blender: smoothies, soups, salsa, ice cream, dips—they're versatile little machines. One of my favorite blender tips: To clean it, add hot water and a few drops of dish soap. Put the lid on and crank the speed up to high. Rinse it out, and it's sparkly clean.

(continued)

- **Zester.** These are around $10, and as I mentioned before, an awesome way to add a punch of flavor to baked goodies, roasted veggies, and salads. (A strand of zest also makes a beautiful cocktail garnish!)

- **Melon ball scooper.** Also around $10, they're perfect for scooping uniform dough balls for amazeballs and cookies.

- **Dehydrator.** This is another splurge option. It's not one I necessarily use all the time but I have definitely gotten my money's worth. A good dehydrator will set you back around $200 but can be used to create raw treats like macaroons, fruit leathers, raw crackers, cookies, pie tarts, and jerky. Many customarily dehydrated foods can also be made in the oven, so while it's fun to have, it isn't a necessity.

Grab-and-go meal and prep plans

To help you get started eating HIIT, I've created four 2-week meal and prep plans, including suggestions for breakfast, lunch, dinner, and snacks. The prep guide includes everything that you can complete on Sunday to set yourself up for success. You can mix and match as you'd like, and if you follow the prep guide, you'll have healthy choices readily available most days of the week. Depending on how many people are in your family, you will have leftovers to enjoy and freeze for later, too.

If you choose to condense your eating period, use these options to create larger meals and eat them within your desired time duration (usually an 8 to 10 hour span). Or, if you find that you enjoy doing mini meals every day, that's great, too! *See what method works best for you and go from there.* As long as you're focusing on whole, clean foods, you should reap the benefits from your hard work. This is the basis of the HIIT lifestyle: prep yourself for success, alternate between work and rest, repeat. Let your intuition be your guide. It will tell you what your body truly needs; it's up to you to listen.

One day each week, enjoy a "wild card" day: an awesome time to enjoy eating out and/or cleaning out the fridge.

A Note on Dinner: If you are cooking for a family, make sure to plan your dinners ahead and make anything you can in advance. If you're cooking smaller amounts for dinner, feel free to repeat lunch ideas or use dinner leftovers from the night before. Just make sure to emphasize protein and produce, especially for your nighttime meal.

The meal plans are split into the following options:

- Omnivore (a little bit of everything)

- Gluten-Free Vegetarian (without fish, poultry, meat, and gluten)

- Vegan (free of all animal products)

- Gluten-Free, Dairy-Free

Omnivore

Week 1

MONDAY

Breakfast: *Breakfast cookie*
Lunch: *Deconstructed sushi salad*
Snack: *Egg and veggie muffins*
Dinner: *Jalapeno turkey burgers with smoky and sweet potatoes*, salad

TUESDAY

Breakfast: *Berry chia pancakes*
Lunch: Leftover *turkey burger* on a wrap or *Thai chicken lettuce wraps*
Snack: *Chocolate protein bars*
Dinner: *Orange honey salmon* with lemon and *lemon and garlic asparagus*

WEDNESDAY

Breakfast: *Breakfast cookie cereal*
Lunch: Chicken salad with *clean Caesar dressing*
Snack: *Egg and veggie muffins*
Dinner: *Chicken crust pizza* and roasted vegetables

THURSDAY

Breakfast: Two eggs wrapped in a tortilla with your favorite vegetables and salsa
Lunch: *Chicken crust pizza* and salad with *clean Caesar dressing*

Snack: *Chocolate protein bars* or small smoothie
Dinner: *Stuffed chicken* and roasted vegetables

FRIDAY

Breakfast: *Baked breakfast cookie* and one egg
Lunch: Leftover *stuffed chicken* and vegetables
Snack: *Chocolate protein bars*
Dinner: Dinner out!

SATURDAY: Clean out the fridge day. Enjoy any leftovers you may have and start to plan for the following week. For the next week, you should still have egg muffins, berry chia pancakes, and chicken crust pizzas on hand.

SUNDAY PREP SCHEDULE:

- Preheat the oven and prepare the chicken crust pizzas (double batch). Allow them to cook while you make your berry chia pancakes (double batch).

- Allow the pizzas and pancakes to cool while you make your chocolate protein bars and baked breakfast cookies.

- Make Caesar dressing to enjoy on salads.

- Chop any vegetables you may need for the upcoming week.

DURING THE WEEK:

- Make shredded chicken in the slow cooker.

- Prepare anything you can the night before (breakfast cookie, set salmon in the fridge to marinate, and stuff chicken the night before, so all you have to do is bake).

Week 2

MONDAY

Breakfast: *Egg muffins* (freezer from last week) OR egg scramble and a baked sweet potato
Lunch: *Quinoa power salad*

Snack: *Low-sugar granola bar*
Dinner: *Slow cooker cashew chicken*

TUESDAY

Breakfast: *Quinoa porridge* with berries
Lunch: Leftover *slow cooker cashew chicken* or wrap (protein, veggies, favorite salad dressing) and salad
Snack: *Amazeballs*
Dinner: *Chicken and sweet potato burgers* with *polenta fries* and salad

WEDNESDAY

Breakfast: *Baked breakfast cookie* (freezer from last week) and an egg
  OR *low-sugar granola bar* crumbled onto yogurt with berries
Lunch: Leftover *chicken and sweet potato burgers* on zucchini or in a wrap
Snack: *Buffalo turkey meatballs*
Dinner: HIIT It dinner combo with grilled chicken, sweet potato, and
  roasted veggies

THURSDAY

Breakfast: *Berry chia pancakes* (freezer from last week)
Lunch: *Buffalo turkey meatball* sub and veggies
Snack: *Low-sugar granola bar*
Dinner: Quiche with *savory butternut squash bites*

FRIDAY

Breakfast: Egg burrito with veggies and salsa
Lunch: Leftover quiche or large *smoothie* with almond butter toast
Snack: *Amazeballs*
Dinner: Out to eat! Order the HIIT It dinner combo (protein, sweet
  potato, and steamed veggies) or something more indulgent that
  catches your eye. Enjoy!

SATURDAY: Clean out the fridge day. Get creative with any leftover produce and take inventory of freezer stash for the upcoming week.

SUNDAY PREP SCHEDULE

- Make low-sugar granola bars.

- While they're in the oven, make chicken and sweet potato burgers

- Prepare the quiche and as soon as the granola bars are finished cooking, put the quiche in the oven.

- Chop any vegetables you may need throughout the week

DURING THE WEEK:
- Prepare anything you can the night before (like the buffalo turkey meatballs and quinoa porridge).

Gluten-free vegetarian

Week 1

MONDAY
Breakfast: *Perfect protein pancakes* with almond butter and maple syrup
Lunch: *Kale slaw with ginger miso dressing*
Snack: *Banana almond muffins*
Dinner: *Marinara veggie bake* with quinoa

TUESDAY
Breakfast: *Homemade grain-free granola* and yogurt
Lunch: Leftover *marinara veggie bake*
Snack: Egg on toast with hot sauce
Dinner: *Sweet potato and black bean chili* with sliced avocado

WEDNESDAY
Breakfast: *Protein yogurt*
Lunch: Leftover *sweet potato and black bean chili*
Snack: *Grain-free granola* and almond milk
Dinner: *Channa masala* with quinoa

THURSDAY
Breakfast: *Banana almond muffins* and an egg
Lunch: Leftover *channa masala*
Snack: *Perfect protein pancakes*
Dinner: Grilled tempeh with sweet potato and kale salad (use leftover miso dressing)

FRIDAY

Breakfast: Small *smoothie* with almond butter toast
Lunch: *Quinoa sushi*
Snack: *Banana almond muffins*
Dinner: Out to eat!

SATURDAY: Clean out the fridge day. Enjoy any last produce you have and start to take inventory and prep for the following week.

SUNDAY PREP SCHEDULE:

- Start a batch of quinoa in the rice cooker to use for salads and as a side dish.

- Prep grain-free granola and while it's cooking, prepare the banana almond muffins and protein pancakes (double batch).

- Cook the protein pancakes and set aside to cool. Bake the banana almond muffins.

- Chop any vegetables you will need for salads and make the ginger miso dressing.

DURING THE WEEK:

- The channa masala is a quick and easy meal you can prepare and enjoy that night.

- For the sweet potato and black bean chili, chop the sweet potato and onion the night before, so the next morning all you'll have to do is add the ingredients to the slow cooker.

Week 2

MONDAY

Breakfast: *Sweet potato breakfast casserole*
Lunch: *Zucchini pizza* and salad with *honey, lemon, and basil salad dressing*
Snack: Apple with almond butter
Dinner: *Quinoa stuffed grape leaves* with roasted veggies

TUESDAY

Breakfast: *Quinoa porridge* with berries
Lunch: Leftover *sweet potato breakfast casserole*
Snack: *Amazeballs* (any flavor)
Dinner: Grilled tempeh with spinach and *savory butternut squash bites* (save half of the butternut squash for tomorrow's lunch salad)

WEDNESDAY

Breakfast: Egg and veggie scramble with sliced avocado
Lunch: *Favorite fall salad with homemade vinaigrette*
Snack: *Protein yogurt* with berries
Dinner: *Warm tempeh salad with mustard vinaigrette*

THURSDAY

Breakfast: *Breakfast cookie dough cereal*
Lunch: *Zucchini pizza* and salad with *mustard vinaigrette*
Snack: *Amazeballs*
Dinner: *Quinoa power salad*

FRIDAY

Breakfast: *Banana almond muffins* and one egg or egg burrito with sautéed veggies and salad
Lunch: *Sweet potato nachos* or salad with protein, quinoa, and fresh veggies
Snack: Small *smoothie*
Dinner: Out to eat!

SATURDAY: Clean out the fridge day. Enjoy anything you have frozen from the previous week, and any fresh produce you have left. Take inventory and start to plan for the following week.

SUNDAY PREP SCHEDULE:

- Make a large batch of quinoa to use for quinoa porridge, power salad and grape leaves.

- Prepare and baked the sweet potato casserole. When you are baking the sweet potatoes, add one or two extras for your sweet potato nachos later in the week.

- Make a double batch of zucchini pizza, allow to cool completely before storing in the freezer.

- Make one batch of amazeballs and store in the fridge.

- Make mustard vinaigrette.

- Wash and chop any vegetables you will need for recipes or salads.

Vegan

Week 1

MONDAY:

Breakfast: *Cinnamon quinoa muffin tops*
Lunch: *Eggplant pizza* (skip the cheese) with a big salad
Snack: Veggies and *chipotle hummus*
Dinner: *Butternut squash mac n' cheeze* with roasted veggies

TUESDAY

Breakfast: *Banana French toast*
Lunch: *Deconstructed sushi salad* (no fish; can add tempeh instead) or leftover *butternut squash mac n' cheese* with veggies
Snack: *Cinnamon quinoa muffin tops*
Dinner: *Warm tempeh salad with mustard vinaigrette*

WEDNESDAY

Breakfast: *Breakfast cookie*
Lunch: Leftover *tempeh salad* and *eggplant pizza*
Snack: *Green smoothie*
Dinner: *Quinoa bake*

THURSDAY

Breakfast: *Grain-free granola* and vegan yogurt with berries
Lunch: Large salad with *tempeh bacon* (save half for tomorrow's breakfast)
Snack: Veggies with *chipotle hummus* or small *green smoothie*
Dinner: Leftover *quinoa bake*

FRIDAY

Breakfast: *Tempeh bacon* and veggie scramble
Lunch: Large veggie salad with *homemade vinaigrette*
Snack: *Grain-free granola and almond milk*
Dinner: Out to eat!

SATURDAY: Clean out the fridge day. Use any produce or freezer foods you may have on hand and take inventory for the following week.

SUNDAY PREP SCHEDULE:

- Make cinnamon quinoa muffin tops.

- While the muffin tops are cooking, make the chipotle hummus.

- Make the dressing you'll be using for the week.

- When the muffin tops are finished cooking, cook the granola.

- Allow everything to cool before storing in the fridge and freezer.

Week 2

MONDAY

Breakfast: *Banana almond muffins* (use a flax egg)
Lunch: *Quinoa sushi* (skip the fish)
Snack: *Amazeballs*
Dinner: HIIT It dinner combo with tempeh (tempeh, sweet potato, and sautéed greens)

TUESDAY

Breakfast: *Breakfast cookie*
Lunch: *Cashew avocado salad*
Snack: *Protein fluff*
Dinner: *Quinoa power salad*

WEDNESDAY

Breakfast: *Breakfast cookie dough cereal*
Lunch: *Kale slaw with ginger miso dressing*

Snack: *Banana tortilla roll-up*
Dinner: *Slow cooker sweet potato and black bean chili*

THURSDAY

Breakfast: Vegan yogurt parfait (layer your favorite vegan yogurt with fresh fruit and cereal/granola)
Lunch: Leftover *sweet potato and black bean chili*
Snack: *Banana almond muffins*
Dinner: *Quinoa power salad*

FRIDAY

Breakfast: *Banana French toast*
Lunch: *Chipotle hummus* wrap (add chipotle hummus to a tortilla and top with your favorite veggies before wrapping)
Snack: Fresh fruit and a serving of nuts
Dinner: Out to eat!

SATURDAY: Clean out the fridge day. Use any produce or freezer foods you may have on hand and take inventory for the following week.

SUNDAY PREP SCHEDULE:

- Start one batch of quinoa for salads and quinoa sushi.

- Bake banana almond muffins.

- Make chipotle hummus.

- Make amazeballs.

- Chop any vegetables you will need over the next five days.

Gluten-free, dairy-free

Week 1

MONDAY

Breakfast: *Blueberry muffin bake* and one egg
Lunch: *Thai shredded chicken lettuce wraps*
Snack: *Grain-free granola* and almond milk
Dinner: *Slow cooker bean-free chili*

TUESDAY

Breakfast: *Grain-free granola* on dairy-free yogurt of choice with berries
Lunch: Leftover *slow cooker bean-free chili*
Snack: Leftover *blueberry muffin bake* crumbled with yogurt
Dinner: *Jalapeno turkey burgers* with *lemon and garlic asparagus*

WEDNESDAY

Breakfast: Two eggs scrambled with veggies and avocado
Lunch: Leftover *jalapeno turkey burger* atop a salad with avocado
Snack: Leftover *blueberry muffin bake* or two egg scramble with avocado, veggies, and salsa
Dinner: *Orange honey salmon* with *smoky and sweet potatoes*, salad

THURSDAY

Breakfast: Shredded chicken wrap (whole-grain tortilla with shredded chicken, mustard, and veggies)
Lunch: Leftover *orange honey salmon* on a salad
Snack: *Grain-free granola* and almond milk
Dinner: *Southwestern Crock-Pot chicken* with roasted veggies

FRIDAY

Breakfast: *Breakfast cookie*
Lunch: Leftover *Southwestern Crock-Pot chicken*
Snack: Small smoothie
Dinner: Out to eat!

SATURDAY: Clean out the fridge day. Use any last produce and take inventory of your freezer stash so you know what to prepare the following week.

SUNDAY PREP SCHEDULE:

- Start the chicken in the slow cooker for your Thai shredded chicken.

- Make blueberry muffin bake and prepare the grain-free granola to bake.

- Chop vegetables for chili and salads during the week.

Week 2

MONDAY

Breakfast: *Sweet potato breakfast casserole*
Lunch: *Cashew avocado salad*
Snack*: Amazeballs*
Dinner: *Southwestern Crock-Pot chicken* with quinoa or brown rice and
   chopped fresh veggies

TUESDAY

Breakfast: Leftover *sweet potato breakfast casserole*
Lunch: Leftover *Southwestern Crock-Pot chicken* on a salad with avocado
Snack: Leftover *sweet potato breakfast casserole* or *protein fluff*
Dinner: *Fish tacos* and *nana's frijoles*

WEDNESDAY

Breakfast: Leftover *sweet potato breakfast casserole* or *easy protein pancake*
Lunch: Leftover *fish tacos* or *chicken spring or nori rolls*
Snack*: Amazeballs* or dairy-free yogurt with fresh berries and honey
Dinner: *Chicken and sweet potato burgers* with roasted veggies

THURSDAY

Breakfast: Leftover *sweet potato breakfast casserole* or two *egg burritos*
   with greens
Lunch: Leftover *chicken and sweet potato burgers* atop a chopped veggie
   salad
Snack: Small *smoothie*
Dinner: HIIT It dinner combo with grilled chicken, sweet potato, and
   roasted veggies

FRIDAY

Breakfast: *Breakfast cookie dough cereal*
Lunch: *Deconstructed sushi salad*
Snack: *Banana tortilla roll-up*
Dinner: Out to eat!

SATURDAY: Clean out the fridge day. Use any last produce and take
inventory of your freezer stash so you know what to prepare the following week.

SUNDAY PREP SCHEDULE:

- Make sweet potato breakfast casserole.

- Prep chicken and sweet potato burgers to store in the freezer.

- Start the chicken in the slow cooker for your Southwestern Crock-Pot chicken.

- Make amazeballs.

- Wash and chop any veggies you will need for the week.

Recipe Directory with Major Food Categories

		Carbs	Fats	Protein	Neutral	Treat
Standby Snacks	Amazeballs, p. 190		x	x		
	Banana Almond Muffins, p. 199	x	x			
	Chicken Spring or Nori Rolls, p. 197			x		
	Chocolate Protein Bars, p. 199	x		x		
	Cinnamon Quinoa Muffin Tops, p. 198	x	x			
	Egg and Veggie Muffins, p. 196		x	x		
	Perfect Protein Pancakes, p. 194	x		x		
	Pumpkin Chocolate Chip Muffins, p. 200	x	x			

		Carbs	Fats	Protein	Neutral	Treat
	Snackable Smoothie, p. 191	x		x		
	Turkey Lentil Muffins, p. 195	x		x		
Breakfast	Baked Breakfast Cookie, p. 208	x	x	x		
	Banana French Toast, p. 212	x	x	x		
	Berry Chia Pancakes, p. 210	x	x	x		
	Breakfast Cookie, p. 207	x	x	x		
	Breakfast Cookie Dough Cereal, p. 211	x	x	x		
	Sweet Potato Breakfast Casserole, p. 213	x	x	x		
Lunch	Cashew Avocado Salad, p. 214		x			
	Deconstructed Sushi Salad, p. 216	x	x	x		
	Eggplant Pizza, p. 217		x			
	Kale Slaw with Ginger Miso Dressing, p. 220		x	x		
	Marinara Veggie Bake, p. 221		x			
	Quinoa Bake, p. 222	x	x	x		
	Quinoa Power Salad, p. 215	x	x	x		

		Carbs	Fats	Protein	Neutral	Treat
	Thai Shredded Chicken Lettuce Wraps, p. 217		x	x		
	Zucchini Pizza, p. 219		x	x		

		Carbs	Fats	Protein	Neutral	Treat
Dinner	Butternut Squash Mac n' Cheeze, p. 226	x	x	x		
	Channa Masala, p. 231	x		x		
	Chicken and Sweet Potato Burgers, p. 225	x	x			
	Fish Tacos with Creamy Lime-Chili Sauce, p. 234	x	x	x		
	Jalapeno Turkey Burgers, p. 225			x		
	Orange Honey Salmon, p. 223		x	x		
	Quinoa Sushi, p. 235	x	x	x		
	Slow Cooker Bean-Free Chili, p. 227			x		
	Slow Cooker Cashew Chicken p. 228		x	x		
	Slow Cooker Sweet Potato and Black Bean Chili, p. 229	x		x		
	Southwestern Crock-Pot Chicken, p. 230			x		
	Stuffed Chicken, p. 232		x	x		
	Warm Tempeh Salad with Mustard Vinaigrette, p. 236		x	x		

		Carbs	Fats	Protein	Neutral	Treat
Sides	Lemon and Garlic Asparagus, p. 238				x	
	My Favorite Fall Salad with Homemade Vinaigrette, p. 238	x	x	x		
	Nana's Frijoles, p. 240	x		x		
	Polenta Fries, p. 241	x				
	Quinoa Stuffed Grape Leaves, p. 239	x		x		
	Smoky and Sweet Potatoes, p. 241	x				

		Carbs	Fats	Protein	Neutral	Treat
Dressings	Clean Caesar, p. 243		x			
	Homemade Lighter Ranch, p. 243		x			
	Honey, Lemon and Basil Salad Dressing, p. 244		x			
	The Best Homemade Balsamic Vinaigrette, p. 242		x			

		Carbs	Fats	Protein	Neutral	Treat
Mini Meals	BBQ Zucchini Chips, p. 246				x	
	Buffalo Turkey Meatballs, p. 248		x	x		
	Chicken Crust Pizza, p. 245		x	x		
	Chipotle Hummus, p. 247	x		x		
	Cookie Dough Bars, p. 251	x		x		

		Carbs	Fats	Protein	Neutral	Treat
	Homemade Grain-Free Granola, p. 251	x	x	x		
	Low-Sugar Granola Bars, p. 253	x	x	x		
	Popcorn Chicken Bites, p. 250		x	x		
	Protein Fudge, p. 255		x	x		
	Quinoa Trail Mix Muffins, p. 254	x	x	x		
	Savory Butternut Squash Bites, p. 249	x				

		Carbs	Fats	Protein	Neutral	Treat
Juices and Drinks	Apple Pear Ginger Saketini, p. 261					x
	Carrot, Apple, Beet Detox Juice, p. 258	x				
	Chocolate Mint Tea, p. 259				x	
	Classic Iced Almond Milk Chai, p. 260				x	
	Classic Sangria, p. 262					x
	Homemade Almond Milk, p. 258				x	
	Iced Coffee, p. 261				x	
	Lucky Irish Girl, p. 263					x

		Carbs	Fats	Protein	Neutral	Treat
	My Favorite Green Juice, p. 257	x				
	Tropical Pink Juice, p. 257	x				
	Tropical Refresher, p. 259	x				

		Carbs	Fats	Protein	Neutral	Treat
Sweet Treats	Almond Butter Chocolate Chip Cookies, p. 266					x
	Black Forest Cupcakes, p. 267					x
	Blueberry Muffin Bake, p. 269					x
	Brown Rice Crunch Squares, p. 271					x
	Cinnamon Apple Tartlets, p. 268					x
	Classic Vegan Macaroons, p. 275					x
	Flourless Dark Chocolate Cookies, p. 272					x
	Mixed Berry Crumble, p. 271					x
	Pumpkin Chocolate Chip Bread, p. 273					x
	Quinoa Cookies, p. 270					x
	Sweet Potato Gluten-Free Brownies, p. 274					x

Foam Rolling Tips

- **Start with less dense rollers and move up.** These are a variety of foam rolling densities, so if you're just getting started, embark on a softer roller. From these you can move up to a dense roller or even the scary step cousin: The RumbleRoller (which has ridges and torture grooves). As you roll each muscle, make sure to hold the tender areas for 30 seconds to one minute. Breathe and think about the muscle relaxing, as it will help to trigger a neuromuscular response in the muscle to actually relax. Our muscles are coated in a layer of connective tissue, called fascia, which can build up and become bundled over time. This can cause discomfort, soreness, and also encourage us to compensate by altering our normal movement patterns. Movement alteration and compensation can lead to injury. Therefore, the foam roller can be a successful technique to maintain full range of motion and protect our muscles in everyday and fitness activities.

- **Do not roll over joints in your body, especially your knees, elbows, or ankles.** Roll leading up to the joint, but never over. Be mindful when rolling your back muscles to keep a straight spine; avoid twisting from side to side, as we have floating ribs that you definitely don't want to roll.

- **This is not a passive technique.** The benefits are similar to deep tissue massage, but here's the deal: you're the massage therapist. This means that you have to do a little bit of work by holding your body weight as you roll. If this places any strain on your wrists, come down onto your forearms or reduce the amount of pressure on your arms by modifying as needed. The more you do it, the easier it will become.

■ **Remember that while foam rolling is definitely uncomfortable, it should never be extremely painful.** If you need to modify by reducing pressure on the roller, please do so! The more you roll, the easier it gets, and the more you'll notice the awesome benefits from this technique.

Some of my favorite rolls

Quads: For this roll, you'll come into a plank position with your hands supporting your body weight. Place the roller underneath your thighs and slowly begin to roll in one direction. When you start to feel a tight spot, hold it and breathe. Take as little or as much time as you need.

Hamstrings: You'll begin this roll seated on the foam roller, with hands behind you on the floor to support your body weight. Walk your hands back to roll down the back of your thighs into your hamstring muscles. This roll is not quite as intense, so if you want to create a deeper release, stack one leg on top of the other to initiate more pressure on this muscle group.

Glute and hip joint (piriformis): You'll start in the same position as the hamstring roll (seated on the roller), but you'll make a figure 4 with your legs by crossing one ankle over the opposite knee. Whichever leg is bent, angle that knee down toward the floor as you slowly roll in and out. This is a killer glute and piriformis roll; awesome for those who do a lot of cardio (HIIT training!!), runners, and cyclists.

Inner thigh (adductors): Come into a plank position, but lower one knee to the floor (so your forearms and knee are supporting your body weight). Place the roller parallel to your torso and your opposite thigh on the roller (bending this leg at a 90-degree angle). Slowly roll in and out, targeting your inner thighs (adductor muscles).

IT band and outer thigh (abductors): You'll come into a side plank position with your bottom thigh resting on the foam roller and your top leg crossed in front and placed on the floor in front of you. Using your foot (the one that's on the floor), you'll guide the foam roller to slowly roll and target your IT band, which is on the outer part of your thigh running from your hip to your knee. Our IT bands can start to get a little sore and achy if we do a lot of repetitive exercise—those repeating the same movements over and over. Runners, cyclists, power walkers: This roll is for you!

Calves: This roll is very similar to the hamstring roll. You'll start seated with your hands planted on the floor behind your hips, and place the foam roller underneath your calf muscles. Lift your hips off the floor (so your weight is distributed between your hands and the foam roller) and start to slowly guide the roller up and down your calves. Need more intensity? Stack one ankle over the other to make things more exciting.

Back (latissimus dorsi): This is a relaxing roll, which is perfect for soothing shoulders that are hunched in office chairs typing or tight from driving. Lie on your back with the foam roller under your shoulder blades, knees bent and feet planted firmly on the floor. Cross your arms over your chest to create more space between your back muscles and slowly start to roll down. This is one roll where you'll want to avoid rolling from side to side. Roll straight down your back.

Back of head: This is another relaxing roll, and especially Zen-like after a long day of work. Place the roller on the floor and rest the back of your neck on the roller, so your head is resting on it (like an awkward, hard pillow). Very gently, turn your head 1 inch to the right to create some pressure on the back of your neck, toward the ear. Come back to center and repeat on the other side.

Chest opener: A fantastic way to end your foam rolling session. Place the foam roller on the floor and have a seat on the very end of the roller. Lie back so the roller is like an extension of your spine, straight on the floor. Let your arms fall open at your sides (like a capital letter "T") and embrace the wonderful heart opener and stretch across your chest muscles. Tight pectorals can cause our shoulders to fall forward and create bad posture. This is a wonderful stretch to ensure that the muscles stay flexible and avoid pulling our shoulders into an uncomfortable position throughout the day. Close your eyes, breathe, and enjoy!

Bibliography

Billat, L. V. "Interval training for performance: A scientific and empirical practice. Special recommendations for middle- and long-distance running. Part I: aerobic interval training." *Sports Medicine* 31, no. 1 (2011):13–31.

Buchan, Duncan S., Stewart Ollis, John D. Young, Non E. Thomas, Stephen-Mark Cooper, Tom K. Tong, Jinlei Nie, Robert M. Malina, and Julien S. Baker. "The Effects of Time and Intensity of Exercise on Novel and Established Markers of CVD in Adolescent Youth." *American Journal of Human Biology* 23, no. 4 (2011):517–26. doi: 10.1002/ajhb.21166

Daussin, Frédéric N., Joffrey Zoll, Stéphane P. Dufour, Elodie Ponsot, Evelyne Lonsdorfer-Wolf, Stéphane Doutreleau, Bertrand Mettauer, François Piquard, Bernard Geny, and Richard Ruddy. "Effect of Interval versus Continuous Training on Cardiorespiratory and Mitochondrial Functions: Relationship to Aerobic Performance Improvements in Sedentary Subjects." *American Journal of Physiology: Regulatory, Integrative and Comparative Physiology* 295, no. 1 (2008):R264–72. doi: 10.1152/ajpregu.00875.2007

Etxebarria, Naroa, Judith M. Anson, David B. Pyne, and Richard A. Ferguson "High-Intensity Cycle Interval Training Improves Cycling and Running Performance in Triathletes." *European Journal of Sport Medicine* (November 9, 2013). Epub ahead of print. doi: 10.1080/17461391.2013.853841

Food and Nutrition Board, National Academy of Sciences, Institute of Medicine. *Dietary Reference Intakes for Energy, Carbohydrate, Fiber, Fat, Fatty Acids, Cholesterol, Protein, and Amino Acids.* Washington, DC: National Academies Press, 2005.

Gibala, Martin. "Molecular Responses to High-Intensity Interval Exercise." *Applied Physiology, Nutrition, and Metabolism* 34, no. 3 (2009):428–32. doi: 10.1139/H09-046

Heydari, Mehrdad, Judith Freund, and Stephen Hugh Boutcher. "The Effect of High-Intensity Intermittent Exercise on Body Composition of Overweight

Young Males." *Journal of Obesity* 2012, 480467 (2012). Epub 2012 Jun 6. doi:10.1155/2012/480467

Lindsay, F. H., J. A. Hawley, K. H. Myburgh, H. H. Schomer, T. D. Noakes, and S. C. Dennis. "Improved Athletic Performance in Highly Trained Cyclists after Interval Training." *Medicine & Science in Sports & Exercise*, 28, no. 11 (1996):1427–34. doi: 10.1097/00005768-199611000-00013

Macdougall, J. Duncan, Audrey L. Hicks, Jay R. MacDonald, Robert S. McKelvie, Howard J. Green, and Kelly M. Smith. "Muscle Performance and Enzymatic Adaptations to Sprint Interval Training." *Journal of Applied Physiology*, 84, no. 6 (1998):2138–42.

Matsuo, Tomoaki, Kousaku Saotome, Satoshi Seino, Nobutake Shimolo, Akira Matsushita, Motoyuki Iemitsu, Hiroshi Ohshima, Kiyoji Tanaka, and Chiaki Mukai. "Effects of a Low-Volume Aerobic-Type Interval Exercise on VO2max and Cardiac Mass." *Medicine & Science in Sports & Exercise*, 46, no. 1 (2014):42–50.

Perry, Christopher G. R., George J. F. Heigenhauser, Arend Bonen, and Lawrence L. Spriet. "High-Intensity Aerobic Interval Training Increases Fat and Carbohydrate Metabolic Capacities in Human Skeletal Muscle." *Applied Physiology, Nutrition, and Metabolism* 33, no. 6 (2008):1112–123. doi: 10.1139/H08-097

Tabata, Izumi, Kouji Nishimura, Motoki Kouzaki, Yuusuke Hirai, Futoshi Ogita, Motohiko Miyachi, and Kaoru Yamamoto. "Effects of Moderate-Intensity Endurance and High-Intensity Intermittent Training on Anaerobic Capacity and VO2max." *Medicine & Science in Sports & Exercise, 28,* no. 10 (1996):1327–30.

Talanian, Jacob L., Stuart D. R. Galloway, George J. F. Heigenhauser, Arend Bonen, and Lawrence L. Spriet. "Two Weeks of High-Intensity Aerobic Interval Training Increases the Capacity for Fat Oxidation during Exercise in Women." *Journal of Applied Physiology* 102, no. 4 (2007):1439–47. Epub 2006 Dec 14.

Wiley-Blackwell. "Better a Sprint than a Marathon: Brief Intense Exercise Better than Endurance Training for Preventing Cardiovascular Disease." *Science Daily* (April 6, 2011). www .sciencedaily.com/releases/2011/04/110405194101.htm

Zuhl, Micah, and Len Kravitz. "HIIT vs. Continuous Endurance Training: Battle of the Aerobic Titans." *IDEA World Journal* (February 2012). www.ideafit.com/fitness-library/hiit-vs-continuous-endurance-training-battle-of-the-aerobic-titans (accessed March 1, 2014).

Index

About the Author

Gina Harney is the award-winning creator of the healthy living, diet, and fitness blog, Fitnessista.com, which has been featured as a top blog in *Fitness* and *Shape*. She is an AFAA-certified fitness instructor, NASM-certified personal trainer, yoga enthusiast, military wife, and new mom. Harney teaches barre, spin, and Zumba classes in San Diego and is a Level One Raw Foods Chef with a certificate from 105degrees Academy. As part of Sage Dance Fitness, she released her first full-length DVD, *Soli Beat*. She lives in San Diego with her Pilot husband, Tom, and daughter, Olivia.

www.Fitnessista.com